212

1277100

OXFORD MEDICAL PUBLIC

PRACTICAL PAIN
MANAGEMENT

PRACTICAL PAIN MANAGEMENT

S. W. CONIAM

and

A. W. DIAMOND

Consultants in Anaesthesia and Pain Relief
The Pain Clinic, Frenchay Hospital
Bristol

OXFORD NEW YORK MELBOURNE
OXFORD UNIVERSITY PRESS
1994

Oxford University Press, Walton Street, Oxford OX2 6DP

Oxford New York
Athens Auckland Bangkok Bombay
Calcutta Cape Town Dar es Salaam Delhi
Florence Hong Kong Istanbul Karachi
Kuala Lumpur Madras Madrid Melbourne
Mexico City Nairobi Paris Singapore
Taipei Toronto Tokyo
and associated companies in
Berlin Ibadan

Oxford is a trade mark of Oxford University Press

Published in the United States
by Oxford University Press Inc., New York

© *S. W. Coniam and A. W. Diamond, 1994*

All rights reserved. No part of this publication may be
reproduced, stored in a retrieval system, or transmitted, in any
form or by any means, without the prior permission in writing of Oxford
University Press. Within the UK, exceptions are allowed in respect of any
fair dealing for the purpose of research or private study, or criticism or
review, as permitted under the Copyright, Designs and Patents Act, 1988, or
in the case of reprographic reproduction in accordance with the terms of
licences issued by the Copyright Licensing Agency. Enquiries concerning
reproduction outside those terms and in other countries should be sent to
the Rights Department, Oxford University Press, at the address above.

This book is sold subject to the condition that it shall not,
by way of trade or otherwise, be lent, re-sold, hired out, or otherwise
circulated without the publisher's prior consent in any form of binding
or cover other than that in which it is published and without a similar
condition including this condition being imposed
on the subsequent purchaser.

A catalogue record for this book is available from the British Library

Library of Congress Cataloging in Publication Data
Coniam, S. W.
Practical pain management : a guide for practitioners / S.W.
Coniam and A.W. Diamond.
(Oxford medical publications)
Includes bibliographical references and index.
1. Pain—Treatment. 2. Analgesia. I. Diamond, A. W. (Andrew
William) II. Title. III. Series.
[DNLM: 1. Pain—therapy. 2. Palliative Treatment. WL 704 C751p
1994]
RB127.C664 1994 616'.0472—dc20 94-21773
ISBN 0 19 262405 9 (Hbk)
ISBN 0 19 262404 0 (Pbk)

Typeset by Downdell, Oxford
Printed in Great Britain by
Redwood Books, Trowbridge, Wilts

Preface

Pain has always been difficult to understand and investigate. The number of people with a congenital inability to feel pain is so small that we can safely generalize and say that pain is a universal experience. However, investigation has been hampered by the fact that pain is subjective and what any one person will feel to be painful at one time may feel more or less painful on another occasion, so even one person's perception of pain is not consistent. Add to that the fact that two people's pain cannot be compared and the measurement of pain becomes a scientific nightmare. Even if it were easy to measure, the scientist would still be confronted by another almost insuperable problem. Volunteers for pain experiments are thin on the ground, and licences to conduct painful experiments on animals are—and should be—extremely difficult to get.

So science has come late to the problems of pain perception. Real development in medicine has always been led by scientific advance. Scientists dominate teaching in medical schools. There has therefore been little teaching about pain. Pharmacologists have taught students about analgesics, but the emphasis has been on their dangers and disadvantages rather than their value. During clinical studies pain has been taught as a tool in diagnosis. Once a diagnosis has been made, then treatment will cure the cause and pain will go. But all too often it does not.

In this book we emphasize the fact that unrelieved pain is a huge problem, poorly understood, and ineffectively dealt with. We seek to explain to clinicians who are not specialists in the management of pain that much can be done by trying to understand the nervous system mechanisms that result in the perception of pain. Pain is always a psychological phenomenon, whether it results from injury, disease, or from no diagnosable cause. Understanding the effect of pain on the mind is vital if it is to be managed as effectively as possible. At the same time, much unnecessary suffering results from a failure of those who have a duty to relieve pain to understand the simple pharmacology of analgesics. Their effective use is too often prevented by lack of understanding of their dangers and the risk of abuse.

We have not written this book as a textbook for specialists or potential specialists in the developing field of pain management. We hope it will be of interest to all others involved in the care of people suffering from pain.

We hope it will challenge some widely held beliefs and be of interest. A more widespread and better understanding of pain and its management would reduce needless suffering and invalidity due to pain, whatever its cause.

1994 S.W.C.
A.W.D.

Contents

1 *The problem of pain*

We have the means and the skills to relieve pain but we do not always use them. Why not? There are several reasons. We believe that other things are more important, we believe that the relief of pain may not always be a good thing, we do not believe people who are in pain, and we believe that it is a good thing to endure pain uncomplainingly.

Then again, pain is not always easy to relieve. The most powerful analgesics have side-effects which can be lethal, and they are abused; the milder ones are not always effective. In some circumstances pain seems intractable, and causes personality changes that increase invalidity and social withdrawal. Some pains are believed to be 'psychological' and thus beyond the reach of nonspecialists. The management of pain is also taught badly—if it is taught at all—to students of the healing professions. This results in many misconceptions.

The result of all these factors is that many people suffer great pain unnecessarily. There can be no higher humanitarian duty than to relieve pain if it is possible. First however we need to understand clearly what it is, where we find it, when it is not being dealt with effectively, and why.

What is pain?

It might seem facile to start this book with such a question. Almost everybody experiences pain frequently and it is often severe. The real purpose of our professional existence is to discover the cause of this and other symptoms and, by curing them, to produce symptom relief and 'health'. As we shall show in this chapter, if health is freedom from distressing symptoms, then medicine has failed disastrously in its principal aim. People feel ill all around us, probably as frequently as they have always done. Modern medicine, complementary medicine and all the developments in the management of human physiology, psychology, and pathology have had very little effect on the incidence of 'illness' in the community. Their successes have been in preventing the spread of disease, and in establishing and eliminating the causes of disease. Common symptoms such as pain remain unrelieved because society equates health with freedom from disease rather than freedom from symptoms.

Much of the pain that is experienced is unnecessary; it is caused by or persists in spite of treatment to cure disease, and results in unnecessary invalidity. This is because we—medicine and society—do not understand pain.

And so we come back to the question 'what is pain?'. It has been defined best by the International Association for the Study of Pain (IASP) as 'an unpleasant sensory and emotional experience associated with actual or potential tissue damage or described in terms of such damage'.

Taking this definition piece by piece we can begin to understand how what pain really is differs from our instinctive conception of it, and thus why we mismanage it. Instinctively we feel that pain is the result of something hurting us. To be hurt is to feel pain and to be damaged, so we cannot escape the belief that pain represents damage to our bodies. We also feel that the intensity of the pain must be related to the degree of damage being done. Thus when we feel pain, we have only two elements in our minds—the sensory element and the tissue damage element.

The IASP definition, however, states that there is an emotional component as well, and of course there is. Pain cannot be experienced without disturbance. This may be annoyance, anger, anxiety, or fear. It may also be the self-control to endure the pain deliberately, for benefit or as part of something desirable.

The definition also says that pain is described in terms of (that is, it feels like) actual or potential tissue damage. However this damage might not exist. Furthermore, actual or potential tissue damage does not always result in pain. Two situations illustrate this. The pain of phantom limb is experienced in a part of the body that is no longer even there, so cannot be damaged. And someone who is hypnotized can undergo surgery without feeling anything. Though these examples are extreme, it is common for us to feel aches and pains where nothing is wrong, and to damage ourselves while distracted by the enjoyment of sport or other activity and not to realize that anything has happened until later.

Thus our instinct says that pain is damage, and that a cure for it must come from healing the damage. Where no damage can be found, or when the damage has been repaired, we feel that pain should not exist; when the damage cannot be repaired we feel that pain is inevitable (see Chapter 3).

Pain and disease as a label

If we are in pain we are 'ill'. Society treats us in an 'ill' way. Part of the response to illness is that other people insist we seek treatment; the sufferer is asked 'why don't you do something about it?' Once treatment is accepted it becomes the imperative. And once treatment is over the sufferer should be better, and have no more symptoms. When the pain continues even after the sufferer has been made 'better', or when the disease is incurable and causes continuing pain, all too often the sufferer is told 'There's nothing more I can do for you'. The situation then becomes apparently hopeless as the treatment of the disease—and therefore relief of symptoms—has been abandoned.

'Useless' pain

A very large proportion of the pains that bring people to seek treatment belongs to this category of useless pain, where there is no actual or potential tissue damage. This category includes 99 per cent of headaches, irritable bowel syndrome (from which 20% of the population suffer), neck and back pain including sciatica, and a lot of chest pain. This does not mean that these pains do not hurt and cause invalidity, that is that they do not cause ill health. It is just that they are not caused by actual or potential tissue damage, so are not amenable to diagnosis of a causative lesion and cure.

Useful common pain

All pain is not, of course, bad. Giving ourselves a headache through over-indulgence in alcoholic drinks teaches us, often repeatedly, that these are mildly toxic, and may discourage chronic alcohol poisoning in some people. Chest pain generated by exercise says that the myocardium is inadequately perfused and oxygenated and that it might be damaged if excessive demands are made on it. Muscle stiffness after exercise obliges us to approach exertion at a rate that our bodies can cope with. Abdominal pain after food controls our excessive eating, while other abdominal pains may tell us that we are dangerously ill.

So pain that informs us that our body has been damaged has a vital function. Together with the sensations of hunger, thirst, and the desire to reproduce ourselves, pain has been an evolutionary imperative.

Pain and injury Pain in our limbs may be telling us that they are structurally damaged and should not be used. It has an important diagnostic function as well. People who are congenitally unable to feel pain do themselves a tremendous amount of damage by continuing to traumatize damaged limbs. Diagnosis of damage and disease may be very difficult or impossible when pain either cannot be perceived, or cannot be described to another person, for example by a paralysed, ventilated patient in intensive care.

This does not mean that analgesia should be withheld from patients whose pain might help diagnosis, as often happens. Physical signs such as tenderness and pain on movement are still present in patients given analgesia to restore their peace and comfort. The organization of modern medicine means that the person who is responsible for final decision making and planning treatment may be the third or fourth person to question and examine the patient. Too often analgesia is delayed until assessment has been completed. The diagnosis becomes more important than the suffering.

The development of pain management

Pain relief and management have been neglected areas of medicine. This is partly because of the way in which our attitude to the relief of pain has developed. Before 'scientific medicine', disease was not understood and symptoms were treated empirically. The rich had the services of trained physicians, who were highly educated men who based their management of disease on an extensive knowledge of classical methods. This often caused the patient a great deal of suffering to no benefit. Sometimes the natural progress of the disease led to a spontaneous cure, in spite of what the skilled physicians had got up to (perhaps little has changed after all).

These remedies were not available to the poor. For them there was folk medicine, which was probably about as effective or ineffective as the physicians' cures. Alternatively there were morphine and alcohol. These did relieve pain and were probably the only remedies that did more good than harm.

With the development of scientific medicine came an understanding of disease, and the possibility of cure became the only proper aim of both physician and patient. Suffering before, during, and often after became incidental. The relievers of suffering—opium and alcohol—became associated with wrong behaviour, and so a belief grew that they were dangerous and should be controlled. This persists today and remains a cause of much unnecessary suffering and misery.

Changing social attitudes towards drugs

Our attitude to drugs that influence mood and relieve suffering remains more influenced by prejudice than benefit and danger. The World Health Organization has suggested that in managing the pain of terminal cancer physicians should push their patients up an analgesic ladder, advancing rung by rung from paracetamol, simple analgesics, and the non-steroidal anti-inflammatory drugs (NSAIDs), to weak opioid–analgesic mixtures, weak opioids alone, and finally to morphine itself only when the pain defeats all drugs below it. There is no logic to this. A very small dose of morphine is no more or less dangerous or undesirable than an equipotent dose of codeine. The reason for the ladder is a lingering belief that morphine is 'bad', worse than codeine or dextropropoxyphene, and should not be given unless the weaker, less 'bad' drugs are not enough. The NSAIDs work in a different way from the opioid group. They should be used alone or in association with them when they are indicated. They are not simply a more desirable, weaker and less dangerous alternative.

Development in cancer pain and postoperative pain

A slow evolution in attitude is now taking place. It started with the changing attitude to analgesia in the terminally ill, pioneered through the hospice movement. Dying patients had been deprived of morphine and other drugs for fear of addiction. But this worry was irrelevant for patients who would die very soon, especially when it meant that they were left in intolerable pain. It was a liberating concept that morphine and its analogues could be prescribed to these patients at whatever dose controlled the pain, with no upper limit. This was the start of a learning process about the use of analgesics which has now spread into the management of postoperative pain. The correct choice of analgesic is the one that relieves the pain, the correct dose is that which does so, and the correct interval between the doses is that which prevents the pain being felt.

The scale of the pain problem

Everybody suffers pain, with the exception of a very small group of people who are congenitally unable to perceive it. It is useful when it detects actual or potential tissue damage. This is not the pain problem. The problem arises when pain persists, and no longer serves any purpose for health and survival, or when there is pain in the absence of any damaging cause.

The science of epidemiology has been almost exclusively concerned with the incidence of disease rather than symptoms, so there are very few studies on the incidence of pain. There have been some studies which have looked at the incidence of pain in the community, rather than more specifically at chronic pain and pain that causes disability. For example, in a survey of 1489 adults in New Zealand (James et al. 1991), 82 per cent of the subjects who responded to a questionnaire stated that they had experienced more than one life-disrupting experience of pain. Crook et al. (1984) looked at 500 randomly selected households in Canada to find out the prevalence of pain. This and the New Zealand survey found that pain was reported more frequently by females than males, and that persistent pain was most commonly reported as arising in the back and head. In 36 per cent of the families surveyed, one or more family members had been affected by pain in the two weeks before the survey. One person in seven (14 per cent) reported a persistent pain problem and 5 per cent a temporary one.

Brattberg *et al.* (1989) looked at the prevalence of persistent pain, its intensity, and its consequences in a single county in Sweden. Two-thirds of the respondents said that they had pain or had had pain recently. In 40 per cent of these, that is 28 percent of the total, the pain had persisted for more than six months. In 58 per cent, the pain was at least as severe as stiffness after exercise. The pain caused difficulties in dressing for 6.4 per cent, and in coping with stairs for 13 per cent of respondents. In 26 per cent the pain interfered with socializing. These relatively small surveys indicate that in wealthy Western communities more than one person in ten suffers from prolonged unrelieved pain.

There have been three national epidemiological studies. In 1985 a telephone survey was conducted in the United States (Sternbach 1986). Ten per cent of the respondents had had joint pain and nine per cent backache for more than 101 days. The writer estimates that in the United States four billion working days are lost each year as a result of pain, five days for each full-time employee. Of those who rated their pain severe or unbearable, 18 per cent had not sought medical advice because they did not believe that anyone could help.

A telephone survey of British households found that 11.5 per cent of the population surveyed had suffered from pain for more than the previous three months (Bowsher *et al.* 1991). Just over half of sufferers (55 per cent) were female, 60 per cent had been in pain for more than half of the preceding month, 55 per cent were unable to work, 17 per cent had retired from work because of pain, and 6 per cent were housebound with pain.

The Office of Population Censuses and Surveys (OPCS) in Great Britain carried out a survey of disabled people between 1985 and 1988. Although this included questions about the incidence of pain, the responses were not analysed at the time—a fact that speaks volumes for the lack of importance attached to the subject. This information has now been extracted and analysed by the Social Policy Research Unit (SPRU) and the results have been both informative and startling. The survey found that 10 per cent of the population was disabled, and of these 41 per cent stated that they suffered from severe pain, 36 per cent that it limited their daily activity, and 28 per cent that it was excruciating, terrible or distressing at its worst. In 6 per cent, the pain was at this level all the time and in 13 per cent it was at least once a day. Pain severely affected normal life in 30 per cent of the respondents.

When the figures were extrapolated, it was estimated that 2 364 000 people suffered severe pain and disability in Great Britain, perhaps 25 000 in the average health district. This study indicates only the incidence of unrelieved pain in the disabled population. Pain in those who are not disabled needs to be added to this total.

The problem then is monstrous. It is present in countries which have been at the forefront in the development of Western medicine and which provide free medical care for all their citizens.

The challenge of pain management

The size of the pain problem is proof that, although Western medicine has solved many of the problems caused by disease, it has not had the same success with suffering.

Analgesics relieve some but not all pain. They only relieve pain temporarily and they do so at a price. The safest analgesics, the least toxic, are the least potent. The more powerful the drug, the greater the potential price in terms of side-effects, dependence, and tolerance. Analgesics are rarely an answer to any pain which may go on indefinitely. Where analgesics are not an answer, other drugs (for example antidepressants and anticonvulsants) can influence pain, but there is very little confirmed evidence of their value and place in chronic pain.

The management of pain is therefore complex. All professionals who care for the sick should understand that pain is still often left untreated unnecessarily. They should know how to assess the extent of pain and how to plan its management. Sometimes the problem is so complex that a specialist in the newly developing field of pain management is needed. But often simple measures are enough, and these are within the capabilities of anyone who can talk to and examine a sufferer, who knows the effects and side-effects of the drugs used in pain management, and who can handle a syringe filled with local anaesthetic.

References

Bowsher, D., Rigge, M., and Sopp, L. (1991). Prevalence of chronic pain in the British population: a telephone survey of 1037 households. *The Pain Clinic*, 4, 223-30.

Brattberg, G., Thorslund, M., and Wikman, A. (1989). The prevalence of pain in a general population. *Pain*, 37, 215-22.

Crook, J., Rideout, E., and Browne, G. (1984). The prevalence of pain complaints in a general population. *Pain*, 18, 299-314.

James, F. R., Large, R. G., Bushnell, J. A., and Wells, J. E. (1991). Epidemiology of pain in New Zealand. *Pain*, 44, 279-83.

Sternbach, R. A. (1986). Survey of pain in the United States: the Nuprin report. *Clinical J. Pain*, 2, 49-53.

2 *The perception of pain*

Pain is unlike any of the other sensory modalities. It is not a single measurable sensation like light and sound; it is an experience, the nature of which depends not only on the nature of the stimulus, but on the programming of pain perception mechanisms and their cerebral interpretation. There is no single pathway in the nervous system which is responsible for the perception of pain. The integrated response of many physiological mechanisms may be interpreted as pain.

The mechanistic view of pain

The seventeenth-century philosopher Descartes proposed that a peripheral noxious stimulus resulted in minute threads being pulled. These threads ran along clearly determined paths to the pineal gland. The mechanism by which the pain message reached the central nervous system (CNS) was therefore similar to pulling a bell cord.

Although the anatomy of the nervous system was mapped in great detail in the next centuries, the essentials of this 'mechanistic' view of pain perception were accepted until relatively recently. Anatomical structures (corpuscles and capsules) were discovered at the endings of some nerves, and specific modalities of sensation were attributed to them. Histological staining of the CNS revealed well delineated tracts in the spinal cord which appeared to have a particular role in sensory conduction. One of these, the spinothalamic tract, was proposed to conduct pain. The specificity theory of pain proposed that certain painful stimuli were detected by specific receptors and conveyed along tracts in the spinal cord to specific areas of the brain where pain was perceived.

However, this system cannot explain:

(1) how pain may return after the cutting of a peripheral nerve or the spinothalamic tract;

(2) why pain may appear to arise from a phantom limb or following a traumatic paraplegia or brachial plexus avulsion;

(3) why pain may develop after damage to a part of the nervous system, even in regions that contain no nerve endings or sensory receptors;

(4) why there may be no pain after injuries received during battle or competitive sporting events, and yet pain may arise long after the painful stimulus has passed.

Controversy raged well into this century between the supporters of the specificity theory and those who proposed the 'intensity theory'. This theory viewed pain as a product of over-stimulation of touch, so that stimulation of a certain intensity for a certain time would cause pain.

Aristotle had originally suggested that pain was an affective quality (a passion), but in the twentieth century it was Sherrington who proposed that pain was composed of both sensory and affective components. The dawn of current concepts came with Noordenbos, who suggested in 1959 that activity in small nerve fibres travelled via the dorsal horn of the spinal cord to the brain, and that when sufficient activity summated, it was perceived as pain. The large fibres, he suggested, inhibited these impulses and therefore prevented summation.

The peripheral system

It is now known that tissue damage, or a stimulus which potentially damages tissue, activates nociceptors (receptors of noxious stimuli) at the free endings of fine unmyelinated C fibres, and larger myelinated A-delta fibres. The A-delta fibres conduct impulses rapidly, from high-threshold receptors for mechanical and thermal stimuli. The C fibres conduct impulses slowly, from polymodal nociceptors which may be sensitive to noxious chemical, thermal, and mechanical stimuli. These nociceptive impulses are conducted to the dorsal root ganglion cells from where they travel mainly via the dorsal root to the dorsal horn of the spinal cord (Fig. 2.1). Some stimuli may travel via the ventral root to the dorsal horn.

Sensory input is modulated at all levels of the nervous system from the periphery to the level of consciousness, and this may enhance or inhibit the perceived sensation. The perceived sensation depends not only on the stimulus but also on the interaction of many other inputs to the spinal cord from peripheral pathways, as well as activity in the CNS and the emotional component of any painful sensation. It is impossible to divide pain between the 'mind' and the 'body'. It is an integrated function of the whole nervous system, including consciousness, and the emotional and behavioural responses.

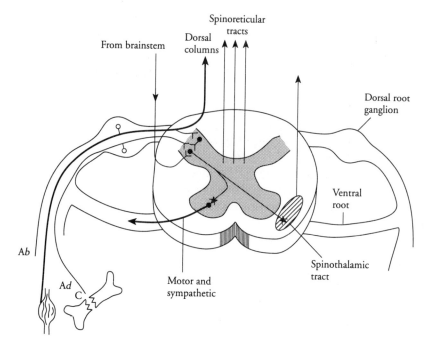

Fig. 2.1   Simplified scheme of nociceptive input to the spinal cord.

At the site of tissue injury, local release of substances such as brady-kinin, substance P, leukotrienes, and thromboxanes changes the physiological environment of the injury (vasodilatation and extravasation), as well as stimulating and sensitizing nociceptors in the area of injury. This results in an increased painful sensitivity of the area.

Central processing

The dorsal horn of the spinal cord is the primary processing system for noxious stimuli. Here, incoming noxious stimuli interact with many other components of the CNS to determine what sensation the person perceives, and so what action results. The cells of the dorsal horn are arranged in a series of laminae. The cells in each lamina interact with other laminae, as well as receiving their own sensory input and descending inhibition or facilitation. The information passed to the brain from the deeper laminae is a complex result of the cascade of interaction between these groups of cells and the rest of the CNS.

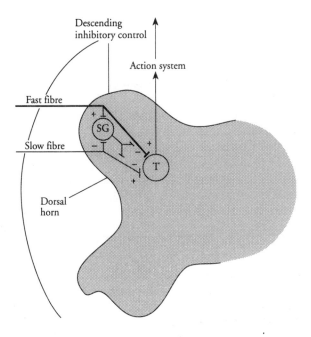

Fig. 2.2 The gate control theory. SG, substantia gelatinosa; T, transmission cell.

The landmark in modern pain theories, the gate theory, is concerned with interactions in the dorsal horn (Fig. 2.2). It was proposed by Melzack and Wall in 1965 and, although it has since been modified, it remains one of the basic concepts of pain theory. Sensory input is transmitted to higher centres by the T (transmission) cells. Activation of the T cells is modulated by a gating system, dependent on the relative activities between the rapidly conducting $A\beta$ fibres and the slowly conducting C fibres. Activity in the faster fibres inhibits activity in the slower fibres. This fits with the common experience that stimulating the skin by rubbing, vibration, or applying rubifacients may reduce pain. The sharp pain following a blow on the shin, for example, travels predominantly in the fast fibres, and is followed by a dull aching pain involving slow fibres. This pain can be relieved by rubbing the sore limb (closing the gate). This idea has been put to practical use in the development of TENS (transcutaneous electrical nerve stimulation) devices for pain relief.

The gate is also controlled by impulses travelling down the spinal cord from higher centres. These descending inhibitory systems appear to originate in the region of the brainstem, and may be activated by the impulses which travel rapidly up the dorsal columns, carrying non-painful and position sensation. The dorsal columns have important effects in the modulation of pain, activating cognitive processes (such as interaction with memories of past events or emotional status, and directing consciousness to other activities), influencing descending inhibition of T cell firing, and so reducing central transmission of noxious stimuli. Only when T cell activity exceeds a certain threshold will it activate the 'action system', the behavioural response and experience associated with pain. When attention is diverted to more demanding cognitive processes, as in battle or sports, there may be a reduction or total absence of pain sensation.

Modulation of sensory input in the dorsal horn involves a large number of neurotransmitters, making it one of the most fertile areas for research into means of influencing pain perception. Peptides and amino acids such as substance P, aspartate, glutamate, and somatostatin are important transmitters in the pain modulation system. Substance P is produced in the dorsal root ganglion cells and then transported centrally and peripherally along the axons. It appears to mediate a slow depolarization of dorsal horn neurones, enhancing the effect of other neurotransmitters.

The descending inhibitory systems influencing dorsal horn activity release noradrenalin and serotonin, and increasing levels of these transmitters appears to reduce pain. This may be the basis for the effects of tricyclic antidepressants and acupuncture. Descending inhibitory systems also involve the endogenous opioids (enkephalins) which interact with spinal opioid receptors and play a major role in the modulation of pain. The discovery of opioid receptors in the spinal systems as well as in the brain stem, has increased interest in the wider application of opioid analgesia.

Central transmission

The modulated afferent stimuli ascend via many pathways. Some travel via rapidly conducting tracts such as the spinothalamic tract to reach the thalamus, and then project to the somatosensory cortex and consciousness (Fig. 2.3). This system conveys rapid discriminative stimuli. Smaller fibres arising from the deeper laminae radiate to the reticular formation, periaqueductal grey, medial and intralaminar thalamic nuclei, and hypothalamus. Some of these tracts terminate near cells which generate descending inhibitory stimuli. Projections to the limbic system and many other areas of the brain influence both the physiological and emotional responses to pain.

Extensive modulation of the pain experience also occurs in supraspinal areas. Anxiety, fear, direction of attention, and cognitive and evaluative activities influence the perception of pain via the descending tracts which modify the activity of dorsal horn cells. It seems that the frontal cortex plays a major role in mediating between cognitive activities and motivational affective features before an integrated motor response is triggered.

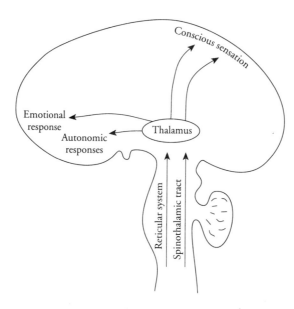

Fig. 2.3 The central projection of pain.

The integrity of the pain perception system

Because the perception of pain is an integrated function of the whole nervous system, no one transmission system can be said to be responsible for the perception of pain. Destroying one tract may modify the perception of pain, but this rarely provides permanent relief. By impairing the integrity of the system, it may eventually lead to increased suffering. Hence, although surgical destruction of the anterolateral spinothalamic tracts in the cord ('cordotomy'), relieves pain for a time, this usually wears off within a year or so. Patients often find that this new pain may be more unpleasant and intractable than the original pain.

Pain may be considered as being physiological or pathological. Pathological pain results from changes in the nociceptive system whereas physiological pain is a result of continual activation of high-threshold nociceptors.

The plasticity of pain perception

The changes that occur in the nervous system associated with pathological pain illustrate that the nervous system is plastic and adaptable, rather than a 'hard-wired' system of circuits. After peripheral injury, an immediate sharp pain signals tissue damage. This is followed by a diffuse deep pain which gradually spreads to produce widespread tenderness and restriction of movement, even if the damage is only localized. It seems that the fine unmyelinated fibres release peptides in the spinal cord in response to injury resulting in long-term changes in the way the spinal cord processes sensory input, so that normal signals of movement and light touch are abnormally processed to produce sensations of pain—the symptom of allodynia.

The receptive field of individual nociceptor neurones in the dorsal horn expands after injury. Repeated stimulation of nociceptor neurones may increase the response of the afferent pain perception systems. This happens through activation of NMDA (*N*-methyl-D-aspartic acid) receptors. It results in 'wind up', when the response to further non-painful afferent stimuli leads to firing in this pain pathway. These changes help to explain why some pain becomes chronic, continuing after the cessation of any obvious tissue damage.

When nerve fibres are damaged by trauma or disease (as in neuropathies) the damaged nerve membrane behaves abnormally. It may present continuous activity felt as paraesthesiae or shooting pains, abnormal mechanical sensitivity, or sensitivity to sympathetic amines as occurs in sympathetic dystrophy. The loss of normal input to the dorsal horn results in an increasing receptive field and a loss of the normal inhibitory mechanisms in nociceptive neurones.

Complete destruction of the nerve root will radically alter the chemical input to the spinal cord. This results in long-term changes in the function of dorsal horn cells, which generate deafferentation pain. The requests of patients, and the temptation of their physicians to 'cut the nerve' frequently meet with unpleasant long-term sequelae.

In summary, pain perception is a complex experience which may be related to nociception or due to altered activity in the nervous system. At every level, that experience may be modulated by afferent stimuli, longstanding changes in neuronal function, and a complex mixture of cognitive and behavioural activities. Descartes' model bears little resemblance to the true complexity of the problem.

Further reading

Fairley, P. (1978). *The conquest of pain*. Michael Joseph, London.
Melzack, R. and Wall, P. (1984). *The challenge of pain*. Penguin Books, London.

3 *The psychology of pain*

Pain as a psychological phenomenon

Pain is felt as potential or actual tissue damage. As a result when we feel pain, or someone describes a pain to us, we seek its physical origin. If a physical origin can be found we accept the pain as real pain. If a cause cannot be found, or the intensity of the sensation seems greater than it should be, then a 'supratentorial' element is thought to have been added. In other words, the pain is in the mind or psychological.

This judgement is quite correct, but not in the way that is intended. Pain is entirely a psychological experience. As part of the development of the gate theory of pain control, Melzack and Wall describe the 'action system' in the brain that is triggered when a noxious stimulus arises within the sensory nervous system and reaches the brain. When activated, this system involves the sensory cortex, which analyses the nature and site of the pain; the motor cortex, where the inevitable motor response or inhibition of response is generated; the limbic system, from which comes the emotional response; and the memory and the special senses. Thus all pain is perceived in the whole aware brain. Without awareness there is no pain. A general anaesthetic removes awareness, no more. An anaesthetized person will respond to painful stimuli by changes in pulse rate and blood pressure, but while there is no awareness, there is no pain.

Rarity of psychogenic pain

When a sufferer complains of a pain which cannot be explained, or when the complaint is greater than seems reasonable, the pain is often described as psychogenic. Pain may result from mental disease, but this is exceedingly rare. This is a common source of conflict between psychiatry and the rest of the medical profession. Non-psychiatrists judge that patients whose pain cannot be explained are mentally disturbed or ill, and refer them to a psychiatrist. The psychiatrist replies that they are not mentally ill. Yes, there is a disturbance of behaviour that is the result of unrelieved pain, but if the pain were relieved the patients would be mentally quite normal. The patients then find themselves diagnosed mentally ill by one group of clinicians and sane by another. The pain is still there.

Factors influencing pain perception

Anxiety and fear

The ways in which the perception of pain can be enhanced or inhibited at various points in the nervous system were described in Chapter 2. Anxiety acts as a facilitator, and can be a cause of pain itself. Expectation of damage has a protective role, by enhancing sensitivity to any stimulation through descending facilitatory pathways, from the cortex to the dorsal horn of the spinal cord. As a result of this the organism functions more efficiently, and minimizes damage through rapidly withdrawing from the potentially harmful stimulus.

This is the healthy role of anxiety. Like many other factors involved in pain, it is beneficial in the short term, but uselessly enhances pain perception long after it could be of any benefit. The prospect of pain—or its presence—generates anxiety. Everyone going to be immunized, going to the dentist, or going to have an operation is anxious, and most of all about the pain that they may suffer. This anxiety can increase the suffering caused by any painful event that follows. It is normal and when contained and controlled does little harm. However, careful explanation can reduce anxiety before painful treatment and as a result reduce pain.

Anxiety becomes more of a problem when the pain itself has become a cause for anxiety, particularly when there is no satisfactory explanation for it—a common situation in chronic pain. Sufferers with diagnosed arthritis, where the cause of severe pain is obvious, are often calm and cheerful, whereas those with low back pain may be desperately anxious and distressed, because no explanation has been provided or, worse still, there are several different, contradictory explanations.

Anxiety generates many of its effects through the release of sympathetic nervous system transmitters, such as noradrenalin, and increasing muscle tone. The increased sympathetic output is itself uncomfortable. The sympathomimetic amines generate anxiety, so a progressive cycle of anxiety increasing itself through its own mechanisms is started. Increased sympathetic tone increases gut tone, resulting in an increased sensitivity to gut activity. Resultant anxiety about abdominal sensation, felt as bowel pain, can become the irritable bowel syndrome (see below).

The increased muscle tone causes fatigue in the contracted muscles at their origins and insertions, and in the joints they move. This in turn causes pain within the muscles and joints, perhaps through ischaemia, or muscle and joint stiffness. There are many theories as to the origin and cause of joint and muscle pains, but none has been scientifically verified. It is however common experience that when a limb is kept under load long enough it will start to ache.

Postoperative pain and anxiety   It is easy for those of us who spend all our time in and around operative surgery to forget the fear and anxiety that it can generate, until we find ourselves as victim. Even then we are like the driver who is being driven. We understand the controls and the rules of the road, we just hope that the team treating us understand them as well as we do. Patients admitted to hospital for the first time are in the same position as we would be on our first trip in a submarine: fearful of the consequences, not understanding the purposes of the actions of people whose hands we are in, and completely unable to influence the outcome of our trip. There is an added element, however. We would not be ill or in pain when we set out on our underwater journey, and the result of the trip would not be painful either.

So the prospect and results of surgery can generate considerable anxiety, fear, depression, inappropriate thoughts, and behavioural change; indeed all the psychological processes associated with pain that we have discussed already.

Simple interventions by all staff involved can reduce these and reduce the pain and suffering associated with surgery. These should start as soon as an operation is being considered. Any doctor or nurse who might need to explain what is involved should bear the psychological effect of what is said in mind. All too often people approach operative treatment with their minds full of misconceptions implanted by people who ought to know what is going to be done, and believe that they do know, but clearly do not. Everyone who is preparing a patient for surgery should emphasize that anaesthesia is very safe, even in the extremely ill, and that modern pain relief techniques mean that pain after surgery can be relieved completely.

Depression and loneliness

Unrelieved pain is depressing and frightening. Comfortable life and pleasure in movement, eating, travelling, and sexual activity are diminished or lost. Sociability depends upon mutual enjoyment to a large extent. Participation in sport, music, and parties is the building block of social activity in young people. They enlarge the social circle beyond the family, and lead to the formation of temporary and permanent sexual relationships upon which the structure of society depends. In the elderly the ability to continue to enjoy some exercise, to leave home to socialize, to travel in comfort, and to relax, to entertain, and be entertained form the basis of social function. The continuing presence of unrelieved pain erodes and then destroys this journey through society.

Unrelieved pain removes part or all of any pleasure, and with this comes depression. Pain and depression interfere with sleep, so unhappiness is added to unhappiness. The sufferer also becomes anxious, increasing the pain and leading to a progressive cycle of deterioration.

Pain resulting from a perceptive disorder

Most of the time we are aware of a very small part of what is happening to any part of our body. Only when we are making use of a part of the body for vision, hearing, feeling or function do we become fully aware of it. The feeling of being in health or unwell must result from a continuous analysis below the level of awareness of incoming sensation. Pain results in a continuous awareness from which there is no relief. Pain overrides the complex system that normally filters what is significant from what is not. Disorder in this system probably leads to pain being experienced. This must be a part of the mechanism by which pain is perceived in a part of the body where there is no lesion.

Abnormal somatic awareness

We can be aware of any part of our body that we choose if we concentrate. Discomfort or pain in an organ will bring it into our awareness. Lack of awareness could be said to be an indicator of normality, health or no pain. When someone becomes aware of a limb, part of the body or organ constantly, this becomes distressing and causes anxiety, which in turn gives rise to symptoms. Palpitation is one non-painful example of this state. Where the subject is abnormally aware of lower bowel sensation this progresses to irritable bowel syndrome, which is painful. There is a barrier that usually prevents the backache we all sometimes feel, the stiffness in the limbs that normally progresses with age, or the common experience of fleeting facial dysaesthesia from generating an abnormal somatic awareness. But when these sensations do progress into prolonged pain they become the most difficult pain conditions to manage.

Pain as a cause of invalidity

To be an invalid is to be treated as someone who is disabled or ill. This can be of value, because medication and rest can accelerate recovery. The help given to people who have been made invalids by blindness, paralysis or other loss of function enables them to live in a world in which they otherwise would starve or die.

Illness excites in the healthy a need to help, which is the root of much that is good in human society. People in pain feel ill. They feel the need of support in the same way as the paralysed, infected or blind person, and this generates the same responses in other people that are evoked by other manifestations of illness.

Learned behaviour

Pain is a powerful teaching process through the essential elements of training, reward, and punishment. Exert yourself when pain is present and you are punished because the pain becomes more severe. Rest, and you are rewarded—the pain decreases. Get up and go to work, and suffer. Go off sick, lie in, and suffer less. Society encourages the adoption of the invalid role. When someone complains of feeling ill, the first automatic suggestion is 'take something for it'. If the complaint persists, then he or she is told to 'see someone', to get medical advice—the second step on the road to invalidism. Reluctance to take something or to see someone implies that there is not much wrong after all. Pain that is being treated is more real and gets more sympathy, more reward. There is no praise for soldiering on.

Thus society encourages an increase in the invalid role and rewards it by an increase in sympathy. The person labelled ill is encouraged to rest, not to engage in household chores, not to lift, and to stay away from work. These are very attractive, especially when the chores are disliked and the work unpleasant. The rewards—the encouragement to learn the invalid role—are very great.

This is not to say that ill people consciously adopt an invalid state to avoid what is unpleasant. The subconscious effect of society's rewarding of the behaviour is, however, that it can generate pain. The complaint of pain, the facial expression of pain, the acceptance of medication, and becoming a patient are all rewarded by a reduction in the unpleasant things in life. Minimizing the expression of pain and continuing to undertake all the activities of a healthy person earn no sympathy.

The uselessness of pain behaviour

An invalid is an individual who is being treated as if unwell. The patient in intensive care, on a ventilator and total parenteral nutrition represents the most extreme example of invalidity. In any circumstance in which activity might cause damage to health, the invalid state has a value. If the lung ventilation of intensive care patients is not supported mechanically they will die; if a patient with a broken leg walks on it, it will not heal properly.

However, in other circumstances invalidism has risks greater than activity. An inactive person is more likely to develop deep vein thrombosis, respiratory infection, and bed sores than an active one. Even if activity soon after operation is painful, it is beneficial. Although the person is being taught by the pain to be invalid, in most circumstances the benefits of becoming active in spite of pain are overwhelmingly greater than the benefits of avoiding activity and remaining ill. The invalid behaviour becomes increasingly valueless to the overall health of the sufferer.

Not only is there a risk of such problems as deep vein thrombosis, but also the invalidity impairs social functioning. The invalid depends on others for care, for financial support. The invalid does not socialize and becomes increasingly child-like, withdrawing from such adult behaviour as sexual intercourse, the leadership involved in parenthood, work, and decision making. This leads to a progressive increase in illness behaviour which becomes progressively inappropriate. This behavioural change is not a rare phenomenon found only in the effete and characterless. It may develop in anyone suffering from an unrelieved distressing symptom, and in particular pain.

Psychological methods in pain management

Psychological method can be applied to all situations in which pain may be experienced. Where pain cannot be relieved by medical intervention it is the only tool left to help the patient cope with the unrelieved pain and the resulting disability. As this book is not intended for specialists in pain management I will simply summarize the methods that a psychologist would use.

Relaxation and hypnosis

Pain causes tension. Tension results in sustained muscle tension and muscle under tension aches. Pain arising in joints causes protective muscle spasm which in turn hurts. This tension and spasm can be brought under patients' voluntary control if they are trained to relax.

When we want to induce relaxation we start from the opposite state of tension. The person is told to screw up the face, clench the fists, tense the abdominal and leg muscles, and to maintain this state for seconds before fully relaxing the muscles. This tension followed by relaxation is then repeated in all parts of the body, from face to hands and arms, to chest, to abdomen, to legs. The sense of relaxation is then enhanced gently by instructing the subject to think of a peaceful situation, to breathe gently, and to sink into a profound state of relaxation and comfort. Inducing a state of peace through suggestion is the foundation of the use of hypnosis in pain management.

Avoiding medical dependency

Treatment is an important generator of medical dependency. While pain is acknowledged as an illness by those caring for a sufferer, the status of invalid—with all that goes with it—is conferred on him or her. The management of pain must begin with every effort being made to provide relief. The next stage must be an acknowledgement by both therapist and patient that no further progress can be made in the relief of the symptom. At this point the role of the medical personnel involved in pain management changes from providing therapy aimed at relief of pain, to protecting the patient from further useless attempts at relief. The sufferer must recognize that invalidity is no longer helpful.

The next step is to analyse where inappropriate invalidity has developed and to change useless invalid behaviour back to normal behaviour. This must be where the doctor withdraws; while there is still a medical presence pain sufferers will continue to seek medical solutions to their problems, to continue the invalid state.

Behavioural therapy

Clinicians who wish to undertake pain management through to this final stage of rehabilitation must work in close collaboration with a clinical psychologist, and understand the way in which clinical psychology produces behavioural change. The patient must understand that the medical process is now over, and the psychologist must be assured that the best thing that can be offered to the patient is psychologically based pain management.

Psychologists help patients to reverse the behavioural changes that have resulted in abnormal illness behaviour. This is achieved by reinforcing a return to normal healthy activity with encouragement, and by stopping the rewards that come from invalidity. Patients are given a progressive exercise programme that has been designed by a physiotherapist to be well within their ability. The domestic and work tasks that are being avoided are analysed by an occupational therapist and the patients are shown how to overcome incorrect beliefs about their ability to perform these tasks. Complaint goes unnoticed, achievement is praised. This sounds simple and in essence it is. However, arranging and achieving such a programme is complex and outside the scope of this book.

Cognitive techniques

Everybody is likely to develop bizarre ideas when they become ill. A famous example is that of the medical student who develops symptoms of each disease as he learns about it. Where a symptom is as distressing as pain, especially when it persists in spite of treatment, these ideas contribute to the pain that is being perceived and the distress that it is causing. Among the most disastrous of these disordered thoughts for the sufferer are the beliefs that the true diagnosis is being kept hidden, that there is serious disease but incompetence has prevented its diagnosis, and that there is nothing left but progressive deterioration and loss of all enjoyment and function (catastrophizing).

At the same time, pain sufferers can relieve a great deal of distress if they can learn to think of the pain in an unthreatening way, to isolate it into one part of the body, or to displace thoughts about the pain with more pleasant thoughts. The skills to do this are learnt from the clinical psychologist and these cognitive therapies play an important part in non-medical pain management.

Pain management group therapy

Sufferers from unrelieved pain are isolated and lonely. They feel that other people do not get into this situation. Psychologically based pain management can function particularly well when patients are treated as a group. The success of the best acts as a spur and a target to the other patients, and they learn just how common unrelieved pain, and the resulting suffering and invalidity are.

Pain management groups, providing group therapy on a psychological base with the aim of rehabilitation are becoming increasingly available. Invalidity is reduced in over 80 per cent of those attending. They cost little, as their principal functions are to reduce drug taking and medication, and to stop the pain sufferer from seeking further medical care, both of which save money.

4 *The assessment of pain*

Pain is a subjective experience, and therefore it cannot be measured by an observer. It is essentially what the person experiencing pain says it is. The expression 'real pain' is meaningless. It suggests existence of pain which is not real, although nobody can describe a personal experience of pain which was not real. We therefore have to accept that when another person complains of pain, it is a real sensation which causes distress. We may consider that the pain described is inappropriate for a given degree of injury or disease. We may feel that the sufferer is not behaving in the way in which we expect someone in pain to behave. We may be unable to explain in terms of pathology why the sufferer is experiencing pain at all, or we may decide that a psychological disorder is responsible for or aggravating the pain. Nevertheless, the pain is a personal experience of the sufferer and we only have that person's description of it.

Factors influencing pain

The assessment of pain must take into consideration the factors which are contributing to it. Pain is a complicated experience which results from input to the nervous system, modulation within the nervous system and interaction with stored information and emotional activity. Each of these factors is important in determining the most effective way of managing the pain.

Nociceptive pain is the easiest type of pain for the observer to understand and appreciate. We know that a recent incision or traumatic injury, the hot painful joint of inflammatory arthritis or the obvious inflammatory changes of local infection are painful. There is usually accompanying tenderness when there is obvious tissue damage and inflammation. However, even in these conditions, careful examination will usually reveal an area of altered sensation (see Chapter 2). Light touch to the area immediately outside the area of injury and inflammatory change is often painful. This cannot be the result of local tissue damage and it demonstrates how changes occur in the nervous system following injury.

The experience of pain following injury varies enormously from one person to another. Patients of the same age, weight, and sex, and having identical surgical procedures require widely differing doses of analgesic to produce the same degree of pain relief. Some of this variation may be due to differences in the distribution and metabolism of analgesic drugs, but there is also wide variation in the degree of pain experienced and the sensitivity of different people to the analgesic effects of drugs. The medical and nursing professions tend to be inflexible in their use of analgesic drug regimens. Doses are based on what the patient 'should' need, and not what they do need. Fixed doses and frequencies of administration are based on tradition rather than observation of patients and their responses to treatment. When the dose of analgesic that we believe to be enough proves to be inadequate to control pain, the patient may be accused of exaggerating it, seeking attention, or even of becoming addicted to the analgesic drugs. Such attitudes are major obstacles to the effective management of pain.

Anxiety is a frequent accompaniment to pain and will increase the subjective distress arising from it. Most people in acute pain are anxious about the nature of their illness or injury, and whether the pain and other symptoms can be controlled. The other discomforts of surgery or trauma as well as the threat to future health or life create anxieties which can make pain seem even more intense. Adequate preoperative preparation, and explanation and reassurance, have a valuable role (see Chapter 3).

The pain of longer term illness, such as cancer, is made worse by fear and anxiety. The recognition of these aspects of suffering is important. Explanation of the symptoms and their management, with reassurance about the control of possible symptoms in the future can allay much anxiety and enable more effective pain control. Help with the domestic, personal, and emotional consequences of terminal illness is an important aspect of symptom management.

Pain scoring systems

Effective pain management requires the assessment of pain as well as the monitoring of the effects of analgesics prescribed. The patient's own assessment of the severity of pain is of paramount importance. After surgery or trauma, a regular subjective measurement by the patient is the most useful guide to the effectiveness of analgesia. It should be routine for nurses to ask patients about the amount of pain they are experiencing postoperatively, just as it is to measure pulse, blood pressure, and temperature. Recording a 'pain score' regularly ensures that those caring for the patient are aware if analgesia is inadequate. By giving the pain a value, they allow the effectiveness of analgesia to be assessed and adjusted accordingly.

The most frequently used pain scoring system is the visual analogue scale. Patients are shown a 10 cm line and told to imagine one end as representing no pain at all, and the other end as representing the most severe pain imaginable. They are then asked to indicate where on the line they consider their current level of pain to lie. The distance of this point along the line can then be compared with subsequent values. As pain is so subjective, and it is difficult to remember previous pain accurately, measurements on a visual analogue scale cannot be reproduced accurately. They are subject to many factors which can bias the score. However, these scales remain one of the most useful means of rating pain and comparing pain levels as they change following treatment.

A visual analogue scale is too cumbersome for regular monitoring of pain for some patients. For patients who are unable to cooperate, a verbal analogue scale is best. The patient is asked to rate their pain on a scale of 0 to 10, or even more simply to rate it as, for example, 'none', 'mild', 'moderate', or 'severe'. These terms can be either charted as such or given values of 0 to 3. The system chosen should be simple for both patients and their carers, as well as indicating changes in pain intensity over a period of time.

Quality of pain

In all situations it is important to determine what type of pain the patient is experiencing. Pain is difficult to describe, but most people give some idea of their pain if given some examples of the types of terms that can be used. Pains described as 'nagging,' 'aching' or 'throbbing' are usually nociceptive, and indicate some actual or potential tissue damage. In acute situations this may be so severe as to be 'cutting' or 'stabbing'. Pain which is like an electric shock or is a 'shooting pain' is often a result of damage or disease in the nervous system. Pain which has a burning quality, with strange unpleasant or painful sensations arising from normal touch, may also have a neurogenic origin. None of these expressions are an absolute indication as to the cause of pain, but they are useful in determining the best treatment.

The assessment of the different components of pain can be difficult. The McGill questionnaire (Melzack 1975) is designed to try to identify and quantify these. It consists of a collection of small groups of words used to describe pain. Some groups describe its sensory qualities (for example, in terms of temporal, spatial, and thermal qualities), other groups express affective qualities (for example, in terms of fear and tension), and a third group uses words to express the patient's subjective reaction to the pain (such as irritating, punishing, and agonizing). The patient is asked to choose one word from each group if it describes the pain. The words chosen help to evaluate the patient's pain experience. Words like 'lancing' or 'shooting' help to indicate a neuropathic type of pain. The use of descriptors such as 'punishing' or 'cruel' may indicate a strongly emotional response to the pain. Numerical scoring systems can be applied to a questionnaire like this to help assess the nature of pain and the response to its management.

It often helps if a clinical psychologist does a more detailed psychological assessment of patients suffering from chronic pain. There are questionnaires to help with some parts of the assessment including that of anxiety and depression, the impact of sickness on patients, and the way in which they see themselves and their pain in relation to others.

Effects on daily life

It may not be possible to measure pain directly, but we can measure the effect that the pain has on various aspects of the patient's life. We can record activities such as walking distance, time out of bed, social activity or work ability, to measure the effectiveness of pain management. Carefully designed questionnaires such as the Pain Disability Index (Tait, Chibnall, and Krause 1990) and The Sickness Impact Profile (Follick, Smith, and Ahern 1985) are used to score the effects of pain on daily activities.

It is essential to assess pain if we are to manage it, but that assessment must include the patient's description of and reaction to pain, the emotional factors contributing to that experience, and the effects that the pain has on the functioning of the person.

References

Follick, M. J., Smith, T. W., and Ahern, D. K. (1985). The sickness impact profile: a global measure of disability in chronic low back pain. *Pain*, 21, 61–76.

Melzack, R. (1975). The McGill Pain Questionnaire. Major properties and scoring methods. *Pain*, 1, 277–99.

Tait, R. C., Chibnall, J. T., and Krause, S. (1990). The pain disability index: psychometric properties. *Pain*, 40, 171–82.

5 Analgesic drugs

Opioid analgesics
Simple analgesics
Non-steroidal anti-inflammatory drugs

Analgesic drugs are generally the first-line approach to managing pain in both acute and chronic situations. They are not always effective, and may have undesirable side-effects which limit their usefulness. An analgesic drug may act peripherally at the site of pain generation, it may affect the transmission of painful stimuli to or in the CNS, or it may affect the way in which painful stimuli are processed in the spinal cord and brain.

Some of the 'simple' analgesics and the non-steroidal anti-inflammatory drugs (NSAIDs) exert at least some of their action peripherally, moderating the chemical mediators of pain generation in the tissues. Local anaesthetics must be regarded as important analgesics, when used to control the acute pain of injury. They are also used to relieve pain in some chronic pain states, when repeated blocking of afferent stimuli to the CNS may reduce a state of continued abnormal activity in the pain perception systems.

At the spinal level and at higher centres in the CNS, opioid drugs interact with opioid receptors to moderate the perception of pain. Drugs such as paracetamol and the NSAIDs also appear to have central analgesic actions.

Opioid analgesics

The term 'opioid' covers all drugs acting at opioid receptors, both the natural opiate drugs like morphine and the synthetic opiate-like drugs such as fentanyl. They are the oldest and most widely used analgesic drugs and provide a standard against which others are compared. They are frequently denied to patients who could benefit from them, or prescribed in ineffective doses. This is partly due to widespread misunderstanding of the nature of drug abuse and also to an unjustified association of abuse with therapeutic use. Improvements in the use of morphine in acute and chronic pain have resulted from advances in understanding of the metabolism of morphine. Improved pharmaceutical preparations of morphine have also contributed to its more effective use.

Over the past 20 years the distribution of opioid receptors in the CNS has been intensively studied, stimulating the search for an endogenous morphine-like agonist. This led to the discovery of the enkephalins and endorphins, the body's own analgesic neurotransmitters. There are several subtypes of opioid receptor—mu, kappa, sigma, and delta have been classified, but the full range is probably more complex. Different opioid drugs have affinity for different types of receptors, and this accounts for their different properties. The analgesic effect of morphine is largely a result of mu receptor stimulation, whereas stimulation of kappa and sigma receptors by a drug like pentazocine is responsible for some of its more unpleasant side-effects. All opioid drugs can cause respiratory depression, constipation, and dysphoria, and all have the potential to be drugs of abuse.

Many patients who receive opioid analgesics for prolonged periods to control pain develop some degree of physical dependence. However, this should not be confused with addiction. A drug addict continues to take drugs for their psychogenic effects and may return to drugs even when they have successfully withdrawn and are no longer experiencing abstinence symptoms. Patients receiving analgesics for pain control may suffer from some degree of abstinence syndrome if the drugs are withdrawn precipitately, but they rarely develop a craving or drug-seeking behaviour. If the pain resolves or is controlled by alternative means, then phased withdrawal of opioids is rarely a problem.

Tolerance—the gradual need to increase the dose of opioid analgesics to maintain a level of analgesia—is probably less of a problem than is often suggested. Patients with painful malignant disease can often be maintained on a constant dose of morphine for very long periods, provided the dose is adequate and given frequently enough. If higher doses are needed it will usually be because of an advance in the underlying disease. If a patient often requests increased doses or more frequent administration it is better to reconsider the dose and frequency than to blame 'tolerance'.

The opioid drugs are commonly divided into 'strong' and 'weak' opioids, on the basis of potency. But both groups exhibit a similar range of side-effects. Codeine (a weak opioid) causes constipation, respiratory depression, and physical dependence, in the same way as a strong opioid such as morphine. However, because codeine is less potent than morphine it will not relieve pain so effectively, while increasing the dose above a relatively low ceiling will result in increased (and possibly hazardous) side-effects. A small dose of morphine will be at least as effective as a large dose of codeine, but with fewer side-effects. However, morphine is shrouded with traditional medical and social taboos, while codeine is not.

Opioid drugs are also divided into pure agonists and those with some morphine antagonist properties—the partial antagonists. Drugs like pentazocine antagonize the action of morphine, but stimulate kappa and sigma receptors, resulting in unpleasant side-effects. Buprenorphine partially stimulates mu receptors although it has some antagonistic action to morphine.

Routes of administration

Opioid analgesics can be administered by many routes. Originally opium was taken orally or by inhalation. With the development of purified morphine, the intramuscular route became the usual means of medical administration. Perhaps this was partly because it limited the use of morphine to the medical profession, but it was also because the oral route seemed to be relatively ineffective. Unfortunately it subjected many generations of patients with severe pain to repeated injections, or to being denied strong analgesics because regular intramuscular injection was not easily available.

The development of palliative care medicine has widened the horizons for opioid use in severe pain (see Chapter 8). Analgesics must be given regularly at an interval compatible with the duration of effective analgesic blood concentrations, and not 'p.r.n.'.

Orally administered morphine is rapidly transported to the liver and conjugated. This means that only about a third of the drug initially reaches the circulation, so the oral dose must be three times the injected dose in order to achieve the same effect.

One of the major metabolites of morphine is a conjugate, morphine-6-glucuronide. This is itself a potent analgesic which has long-lasting effects. With regular morphine administration the metabolic products accumulate, resulting in enhanced analgesia. This is the reason that a single dose of oral morphine may provide poor analgesia, whereas regular doses may result in satisfactory analgesia.

Because of its acceptability to patients, and ease of administration, the oral route is the method of choice for long-term analgesic drug administration. Patients who are unable to take oral medication, or who need rapid pain relief should be given morphine by other routes.

The analgesic effect of an intravenous injection is rapid and predictable, so this is the best route for acute post-traumatic pain. The effect can be assessed by both patient and doctor or nurse so that the dose can be titrated against the patient's pain with repeated increments. This is the principle behind patient-controlled analgesia (PCA). Satisfactory analgesia for continuing severe pain may need an intravenous infusion of morphine in order to maintain stable plasma levels.

Another method of producing continuous analgesia is a subcutaneous infusion. This is suitable for debilitated patients receiving palliative care who are unable to take and absorb large quantities of opioids orally, and in whom continuous intravenous access is not needed. The drug of choice is diamorphine, where it is available for medical use (see p. 31). It is very soluble and it is therefore possible to administer large doses in very low volumes by the subcutaneous route.

Opioids can also be given rectally. Morphine or oxycodone suppositories provide long-lasting analgesia which largely avoids rapid uptake and metabolism of the drug by the liver. Patients unable to take oral drugs, perhaps because of vomiting, can continue opioid analgesia in this way. An oxycodone suppository at night can provide a pain-free night's sleep.

Buprenorphine and phenazocine can both be given sublingually. In fact, buprenorphine must be given by this route as swallowing it will inactivate it. Many patients prefer this way of taking oral medication if they find tablets difficult to swallow.

Transdermal delivery of opioids by skin patches has been developed and is likely to become more widely available in the future.

The discovery of opioid receptors in the spinal cord led to the development of the epidural and spinal routes of administration of opioid drugs. By injecting morphine into the epidural space it is possible to produce intense long-lasting analgesia. Only small doses are necessary (1–5 mg) to produce much more intense analgesia than can be obtained with a larger dose given systemically, because the drug acts directly on the spinal receptors. Good analgesia can be obtained without stimulating central receptors, so avoiding many of the side-effects of opioids. Epidural opioids produce the same qualitative analgesia as by other routes. They relieve continuous aching pain but, unlike local anaesthetics, they do not prevent the sharp pain of injury or movement of injured tissue. Local anaesthetics and opioids can be effectively combined in epidural administration (see Chapter 7).

The uses of different analgesic drugs will be discussed in the appropriate sections later in this book, but some general points about the commonly available analgesics will be described at this stage.

Morphine

As with all the strong opioid analgesics, morphine is most effective in controlling severe pain arising from trauma, acute visceral pain, and pain arising in many types of cancer. It is effective in musculoskeletal pain although it will not prevent 'incident' pain—the sharp type of pain that arises on moving a fractured long bone, or coughing after a thoracotomy. Its use may be occasionally justified in the long-term management of severe musculoskeletal pain if this is shown to be responsive to morphine and if all other means of controlling the pain have been proved inadequate.

Unfortunately most chronic pain of this type does not seem to be very responsive to morphine. Chronic pain has a complex aetiology and rarely can one simple analgesic manage it adequately. Pain resulting from damage to or malfunctioning of nervous tissue (neurogenic or neuropathic pain) is usually unresponsive or only poorly responsive to morphine. Examples of this type of pain are trigeminal neuralgia, post-herpetic neuralgia, post-stroke pain, and phantom limb pain. It is important to determine whether a pain is responsive to morphine (even though this may require a higher dose than we have been conditioned to accept as 'normal'). If there is a beneficial response it is logical to continue with this type of analgesia. In these circumstances psychological dependence is rare. Continued administration of morphine for non-responsive pain usually results in undesirable side-effects.

When pain is responsive to morphine but the drug is administered in inadequate doses or too infrequently, patients may continue to request an increasing amount. This is not proof of addiction, and an appropriate dose regimen may prevent this reasonable 'drug-seeking behaviour'.

A single dose of morphine may be expected to provide three to four hours of analgesia, although there can be considerable individual variation in drug handling between patients. Thus, morphine should be given regularly every three or four hours. A longer interval allows plasma levels to fall unacceptably, resulting in a return of pain. Effectiveness of the drug is improved and side-effects minimized when plasma levels are kept constant.

If patients are being maintained on regular oral morphine then in most situations it is preferable to give a slow-release preparation, rather than standard morphine elixir or tablets every three to four hours. The same total 24 hour dosage as is effective when given four hourly can be given in two 12-hourly doses of sustained-release morphine. 'Continus' tablets are designed to release the drug over a 12-hour period. If analgesia appears to be inadequate then it is better to increase the dose than the frequency of administration, as this can lead to accumulation. Doses should never be given at intervals of less than eight hours. Sustained-release morphine is not suitable for the control of acute severe pain.

Diamorphine

Diamorphine is unavailable for medicinal use in most countries where legal restrictions attempt to curb abuse of this drug. In Britain, it is available and widely used in palliative care. It is metabolized to morphine, but has some valuable differences. It is claimed to have a more rapid onset of action than morphine, although this is unlikely to make a significant clinical difference. Its main advantage is its high solubility. This means that large doses can be delivered subcutaneously in a small volume, for instance in the control of pain in advanced malignant disease, allowing greater absorption and comfort for the patient.

The lipid solubility of diamorphine makes it one of the most suitable opioid drugs to deliver via the epidural route (see Chapter 7).

Methadone

Methadone has long been used for reducing consumption of other opioids by addicts. It is also a potent cough suppressant. And it is a useful analgesic, which is often tolerated orally by patients who are unable to tolerate morphine. It also has a long period of action which is useful for management of pain in malignant disease, when a six- or eight-hourly dose regimen is usually effective. However, methadone has a cumulative sedative effect and response must be carefully monitored, especially in the elderly.

Pethidine

When pethidine was introduced it was hoped it would have less abuse potential than morphine. Unfortunately, because of its relatively short action (two or three hours), it may be more likely to result in drug-seeking behaviour. Together with the fact that it can produce all the unpleasant side-effects of other opioids, especially nausea and dizziness, this makes it an unsuitable drug for management of long-term pain.

Pethidine has a higher oral bioavailability than morphine and so has some popularity by this route. It is also claimed to have less effect on smooth muscle, so for many specialists it is the analgesic of choice for managing the short-term pain of biliary and renal colic.

Phenazocine

This drug is well absorbed by the sublingual route, is less sedating than morphine, and its effects last for about six hours. It is therefore a useful alternative in the management of opioid-sensitive chronic pain if morphine is not tolerated.

Buprenorphine

Buprenorphine is well absorbed sublingually and is also available in injectable form. It is a partial agonist which stimulates the mu receptors but binds to them very firmly. It has a long period of action, usually lasting six to eight hours. These factors seem to make it useful in the postoperative period when a progression from injection to tablet can be made. However, its use has been limited by a high incidence of nausea and vomiting as well as dizziness, which are more prominent in ambulant patients. The drug also has a low dose–effect ceiling, so increasing the dose above this level does not significantly increase the analgesia, but may lead to respiratory depression which is relatively insensitive to reversal by naloxone. Some patients with severe chronic pain (for example with ischaemic limb disease) do tolerate the drug well and find it valuable.

Dipipanone

Dipipanone is only available in a combination with cyclizine (dipipanone 10 mg plus cyclizine 30 mg). It is a potent analgesic, with an action lasting three to four hours. However, increasing the dose of opioid increases the dose of cyclizine, resulting in excessive drowsiness. The combination is also commonly associated with drug-seeking behaviour due partly to its short activity and partly to the fact that it seems to produce a slight euphoriant effect in some people. It is not generally recommended for long-term use.

Dextromoramide

This is a potent analgesic, and is perhaps less sedating than morphine, but its short period of action limits its use for regular analgesia. It is sometimes used in patients with malignant disease who are taking long-acting analgesics, but occasionally need extra analgesia, for example during predictably painful daily activities.

Codeine and dihydrocodeine

Codeine phosphate is a weak opioid drug. It slows down gastrointestinal passage, and is widely used as an analgesic. At recommended doses it is relatively weak, but attempts to increase the dose result in excessive side-effects of sedation, dizziness, respiratory depression, and constipation, without useful increases in analgesia. Dihydrocodeine has similar properties. They are both frequently prescribed in fixed dose combination with paracetamol where there may be some advantages. Codeine is traditionally used after intracranial surgery in the belief that it produces less respiratory depression or masking of vital signs than more potent opioids. However, there is little firm evidence that at equianalgesic doses (which are not necessarily achievable) its side-effects are less. The codeine drugs can induce a degree of physical dependence.

Combinations of paracetamol 500 mg with codeine phosphate (8 mg as in co-codamol or 30 mg as in Tylex and Solpadol) are popular and useful analgesics in acute postoperative or traumatic pain, and in longer-term pain such as degenerative musculoskeletal conditions or headache. Dihydrocodeine is available in similar combination (10 mg dihydrocodeine in co-dydramol). Recently combinations of codeine with NSAIDs such as ibuprofen have become available.

It is possible that combining analgesics with different modes of action, can improve analgesia in some situations. However, different lengths of action may mean that a combined preparation cannot be given at intervals suitable for both components, and they may be better given separately. Patients particularly need to be warned not to exceed the safe dose of paracetamol (see Chapter 7).

Codeine drugs are available as soluble or liquid formulations which many patients find more acceptable than tablets. A slow-release preparation of dihydrocodeine (60 mg as DHC Continus) provides a 12-hourly dose regimen for longer-term management of pain.

Simple analgesics

There is nothing particularly simple about the drugs collected under this heading but they include analgesics which are not opioids and are not specifically described as anti-inflammatory drugs.

Aspirin

Aspirin and the salicylic acid derivatives were the first 'modern' analgesics. Aspirin's use as an antipyretic and anti-inflammatory made it an important drug in the early days of industrial pharmaceuticals. It has mild analgesic activity and is useful in mild trauma and headache. As an anti-inflammatory, it was widely used in the management of rheumatic diseases. It is often combined with paracetamol. It is also combined with opioid drugs such as papaveretum or morphine, enhancing their analgesic effects when there is an inflammatory component to the pain.

Use of aspirin, however, has declined because of its adverse effects:

(1) its anti-platelet activity, which increases bleeding after trauma;
(2) its irritant effect on gastric mucosa, and high incidence of GI bleeding;
(3) its association with the rare Reye's syndrome in children.

It is therefore unsuitable for patients with a history of peptic ulceration, and its use in children has been proscribed. Its effect on platelet function has led to its modern use as a prophylactic to reduce the incidence of coronary thrombosis.

Paracetamol

This has become the most popular analgesic and antipyretic for self-medication for all types of mild pain, including trauma, headache, and abdominal pain, as well as the pyrexia and malaise that accompany infections such as colds and flu. It is extremely safe when taken in the correct dose, but exceeding the dose can result in irreversible liver damage. Paracetamol has completely replaced aspirin as the analgesic and antipyretic for use in children, and its availability as a pleasant tasting elixir and as suppositories makes it almost universally acceptable. It has no anti-inflammatory activity but it may be combined with an anti-inflammatory drug. It is also frequently combined with a mild opioid such as codeine or dihydrocodeine.

Nefopam

Nefopam is chemically unrelated to other analgesics. It is occasionally useful in the management of musculoskeletal pain and headache in patients who are intolerant of opioids or NSAIDs. Its use sometimes results in sweating, nausea, and urinary retention. Caution should also be exercised where there is any impairment of hepatic function. Nevertheless, it is worth considering when little else seems acceptable to the patient. It is moderately potent at doses of 30–90 mg taken orally three times a day.

Non-steroidal anti-inflammatory drugs

NSAIDs were developed for the management of musculoskeletal pain, especially in the arthritic diseases. They exert their potent effects predominantly by inhibiting synthesis of prostaglandins involved in the inflammatory process following tissue trauma and in inflammatory disease. This reduces pain at the site of trauma and inflammation. NSAIDs may also affect some of the other chemical mediators of the inflammatory process, and some may have more direct analgesic activity.

All NSAIDs have side-effects which may restrict their use. The reduction of prostaglandin synthesis makes the gastrointestinal mucosa more susceptible to erosion, and the drugs should be avoided in patients with a recent history of peptic ulceration. The effects on prostaglandins can also adversely affect renal function and NSAIDs should be used with great caution if there is any suspected impairment of renal function. Reduction of platelet function makes patients more prone to prolonged bleeding after trauma. Occasional NSAIDs cause severe hypersensitivity reactions, and they are best avoided in asthmatic patients.

NSAIDs are some of the most frequently prescribed drugs, and there are many different drugs available. There are only small differences between them and the most important consideration in prescribing decisions is probably the physician's familiarity with the drugs. Small differences in potency or incidence of side-effects are often promoted by the pharmaceutical companies, but the effect of all these drugs is much the same: they provide analgesia for mild to moderate pain, and are especially effective where there is an element of inflammatory pain and tissue trauma. They are widely used in arthritis, but they do not appear to affect the natural course of the disease process.

Differences in preparation are perhaps more important than the chemical differences between NSAIDs. Although their effect on the gastric mucosa is largely a systemic effect, enteric-coated preparations or suppositories may cause less local irritation and allow the drug to be tolerated in some patients who otherwise suffer from unacceptable gastrointestinal effects. Soluble and slow-release preparations also extend their versatility.

The introduction of injectable NSAIDs has promoted their use in the postoperative period and acute trauma. The parenteral preparation of diclofenac has been available for some time, but its potential was slow to be developed. The injection is not suitable for intravenous use and the intramuscular injection is painful and results in some muscle damage. The development of ketorolac—which does not have these disadvantages— has encouraged further use of NSAIDs. Diclofenac can be given as a suppository before or immediately after surgery, or ketorolac can be given intra- and post-operatively. They enhance postoperative analgesia produced by opioid drugs, and are sufficiently potent to make opioid analgesics unnecessary after some types of surgery, or at least to greatly reduce the requirement for opioids (morphine-sparing effect). This minimizes the undesirable side-effects of opioids whilst improving analgesia. NSAIDs can be particularly useful following orthopaedic and dental surgery, or any surgery that involves extensive musculoskeletal trauma. In some situations where postoperative pain is not adequately controlled with opioids, the addition of a NSAID will result in satisfactory control.

Several anti-inflammatory drugs have become available as topical preparations. Benzydamine, piroxicam, and diclofenac are available as creams or gels to ease the pain and inflammation associated with soft tissue trauma. Benzydamine oral rinse alleviates oropharyngeal inflammation and pain associated with infection or following radiotherapy.

6 *Stimulation to relieve pain*

Transcutaneous electrical nerve stimulation
Acupuncture
Further reading

The development of scientific medicine meant that efforts to relieve pain were concentrated on the pharmacological approach, or attempts to block the neuronal pathways associated with pain using local anaesthetics or destructive lesions. However, older methods of treating pain and disease—including acupuncture, electric shock, vibration and massage, poultices, and painful stimuli such as cupping and scarifying—had aimed at stimulating part of the nervous system. Because such methods could not be explained by the scientific knowledge of the last century, they generally fell out of favour with the medical establishment. These techniques became more or less confined to 'alternative' or 'complementary' practitioners.

Modern understanding (so far as it goes) of the pain perception systems has led to a reconsideration of stimulatory techniques. Rubbing an injured part of the body can relieve pain. Liniments providing chemical stimulation, poultices, and heat lamps are commonly used to ease muscular aches and pains. Stimulation of some types of nerves (mainly the rapidly conducting $A\beta$ fibres) will reduce input by smaller $A\delta$ and C fibres to the CNS. This is the basis of the gate theory of pain (see Chapter 2).

Many of these old methods of pain relief act by stimulating low-threshold mechanoceptors in the skin and subcutaneous tissues, thus blocking input from the nociceptive fibres. The alternative practitioners were exploiting this idea long before the gate theory was conceived.

Transcutaneous electrical nerve stimulation

Techniques of stimulation therapy have been refined to be less unpleasant or potentially damaging than some of the traditional methods. Transcutaneous electrical nerve stimulation (TENS) was designed to provide an effective form of stimulatory analgesia. Patients use a device that generates an electrical wave form and transmits it via conducting electrode pads to the skin. This relieves many types of pain, from chronically painful conditions to the pain of childbirth and postoperative pain.

The pulse generator is contained in a box approximately the size of a cigarette packet (Fig. 6.1). It is battery operated, and a long-life battery usually lasts for around 70 hours. Some models incorporate a rechargeable power pack.

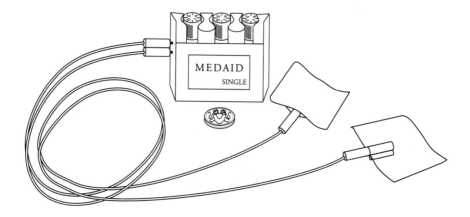

Fig. 6.1   Transcutaneous nerve stimulator.

The pulse generated may be biphasic, sinusoidal or square wave, but there is a trend towards the use of a square wave, as this appears to be the most comfortable form of stimulation. The pulses may be delivered as a continuous train of stimuli or in bursts, and the amplitude may be modulated to produce 'ramped' stimulation. These different modes of stimulation are designed to enhance analgesia. Bursts of stimuli may not only produce TENS analgesia but also recruit other forms of analgesia more akin to that produced by acupuncture (see p. 41). The different modes may also help to reduce the attenuation of analgesia that often occurs with prolonged use of TENS.

Impulses are applied to the skin through electrodes—usually small rectangular pads of carbonized silicone rubber. Electrical contact is made by applying a conductive gel to the pads and then securing them to the skin with adhesive tape. Alternatively, a conductive adhesive gel can be used, to avoid the need for tape. Occasionally patients develop a skin sensitivity to the electrodes or the gel. In these cases it is preferable to use a self-adhesive karya gum electrode. Although these are more expensive and have a more limited life, they are well tolerated.

Some time should be spent explaining the technique of TENS to the patient, demonstrating correct use of the device, suggesting appropriate positions for the electrodes, and advising on how to gain the most benefit from the system.

The electrodes are usually applied proximally over the course of the cutaneous nerve supply to the region of pain. It is important that the electrodes are placed over skin which has an intact nerve supply, as the stimulus should pass up intact large sensory fibres. If the painful area is numb (as may occur following nerve damage) then the electrodes must be placed over the normal skin proximal to this area. Usually, the closer together the pads are placed, the more intense the stimulation, although sometimes it is necessary to stimulate areas quite far apart. The electrodes must not be in contact with each other.

The best position for the electrodes is found by experiment, and the patient must be encouraged to alter their positions to achieve the best effect. In some situations anatomical considerations determine the optimum position for the electrodes. In childbirth it is necessary to stimulate the lower thoracic dermatomes in the first stage of labour. As labour progresses to the second stage and the pain is largely conducted via the sacral nerves, then the electrodes are moved lower down the back to lie over the sacral dermatomes. For managing back pain then it is usually best to position the electrodes over the skin immediately lateral to the spine in the painful region. Claims have been made that good results can be obtained by locating electrodes over traditional acupuncture points.

Once the electrodes have been applied the device is switched on, and the amplitude is slowly increased until the patient reports a definite but not painful tingling sensation. The pulse width can be varied on most models of stimulator, usually between 50 and 200 microseconds. Too short a pulse fails to produce stimulation at comfortable amplitudes, whereas too wide a pulse produces undesirable current and heat. Again, the patient should be encouraged to experiment to find the most comfortable pulse width.

The rate of stimulation may be varied from 2 to 200 Hz. The low rates probably produce analgesia partly by an effect similar to acupuncture, and this may be achieved with some devices by using short bursts of stimuli. After experimenting, most patients find that a frequency in the range of 50–100 Hz is most effective, producing a comfortable tingling sensation.

Some patients with chronic pain conditions choose to use their stimulator at the times when they most need relief. This may be during periods of maximal activity, or after the day's activity when they are trying to relax. Others prefer to use it continuously.

TENS has no known curative value, although many patients experience prolonged relief after ceasing stimulation. However, with some types of musculoskeletal pain, the relief provided by TENS may allow stiff, painful muscles a greater range of movement and thereby gradually improve the underlying condition.

Many patients benefit from a period without their TENS for a few days every month. Apart from acting as a trial to determine whether TENS is still of benefit to that individual, this may help to prolong its effectiveness. After a year only about 30 per cent of those who initially benefited continue to do so. The initial potent placebo effect of TENS is not maintained, but there does also seem to be some genuine physiological attenuation of the analgesic effect in some people.

The indications for TENS are:

(1) acutely painful conditions, particularly where reducing analgesic medication is desirable (for instance during labour or postoperatively in patients with respiratory insufficiency);

(2) somatic pain arising from painful muscles and joints (as in chronic back pain);

(3) neurogenic pains such as post-herpetic neuralgia may respond to TENS.

Pain without any apparent cause often does not respond well. It is obviously necessary to have good patient compliance for TENS to be effective, and the patient must also be physically capable of applying the electrodes, or must have assistance readily available. The electrodes should not be applied to the anterior of the neck, as stimulation of the carotid sinus may result. TENS is not suitable for use by patients with cardiac pacemakers, by those who develop an allergy to the electrodes, or in early pregnancy.

Although some capital investment is necessary for TENS, the long-term costs compare favourably with drug regimens, and the side-effects are likely to be far less troublesome.

Acupuncture

Acupuncture is one of the oldest systems of medicine. The first treatise on acupuncture was written by the Yellow Emperor in China, more than 2000 years ago. The traditional systems practised in the Far East evolved into complex and comprehensive systems for the diagnosis and treatment of most common ailments. Traditional acupuncture proposes that the vital energies of life—the 'Yin' and the 'Yang' which occur throughout the universe—are also represented in the organ systems of the body. The balance between these two forces is essential for good health, and is dependent on the flow of energy, or 'chi', in channels throughout the body. Imbalance results in disease, and acupuncture restores health by promoting the flow of chi and restoring the balance. This is achieved by stimulating the body tissues at certain acupuncture points which lie along the channels, or meridians. Diagnosis involves a complex analysis of the pulses.

Acupuncture has developed along two separate but at times convergent paths. Traditional acupuncture maps many hundreds of acupuncture points over the body surface, and many proponents of acupuncture claim that good results are only possible by stimulating accurately located points. The points chosen to treat a painful condition will generally be a combination of points which lie over tender areas, and more distant points which lie on meridians passing through the area of pain. However, many modern practitioners only use tender 'trigger points' for stimulation, regardless of whether these are traditional acupuncture points. Effective relief of pain can be obtained with both methods and there are probably advantages of combining the two approaches. Little is known about the effects of acupuncture on symptoms other than pain and they will not be considered further here.

In Western medicine, acupuncture is most commonly used for musculo-skeletal pain (Chapter 10).

Possible mechanisms

To minds trained in Western medicine with its emphasis on scientific proof, traditional acupuncture sounds totally irrational. We therefore cannot believe that it can possibly accomplish the mystical and unscientific claims made for it. The life forces cannot be demonstrated by any scientific method and the meridians cannot be demonstrated anatomically. However, the apparent successes of acupuncture began to interest the Western world in this century and it became a popular form of alternative medicine from the 1960s onwards. In more recent years acupuncture has been more carefully examined by the medical establishment. Research in China and the West has begun to show a scientific explanation for some aspects of acupuncture: just because the traditional explanations are unacceptable to most Western doctors, there is no reason to assume it does not work. Acupuncture in the West has begun to evolve from a mystical fringe practice of dubious worth into an interesting and useful tool in the analgesic armamentarium. Its fascinating mode of action is gradually being discovered.

The level of enkephalins in cerebrospinal fluid (CSF) increases after some types of acupuncture. It is also possible that different enkephalins are released in response to different types of acupuncture stimulation. Further evidence for their role is that acupuncture analgesia is reduced by naloxone, which blocks opioid receptors.

Electrical stimulation of areas in the mid-brain, such as the periaqueductal grey and the nucleus raphe magnus, can produce quite profound analgesia which appears to be mediated by endogenous opioids. This is one way in which stimulation can produce analgesia. Long periods of intense manual or electrical stimulation of acupuncture points produce intense analgesia. This technique has been used to produce surgical analgesia which seems to be naloxone reversible.

Brief stimulation of trigger points, as used in the treatment of musculo-skeletal problems, appears to have a different mode of action. Many transmission systems in the nervous system seem to be affected by acupuncture and many different neurotransmitters involved. It seems likely that descending inhibitory tracts in the spinal cord play a role in acupuncture analgesia, and the effect is bilateral—stimulation of one side of the body can produce analgesia in the opposite side. Drugs which enhance these systems of inhibition offer opportunities for enhancing acupuncture analgesia. Acupuncture can produce prolonged analgesia, which may be a result of the stimulation of reverberating pathways within the CNS and hence continued activation of endogenous inhibitory systems.

Further reading

Baldry, P. E. (1989) *Acupuncture, trigger points and musculoskeletal pain.* Churchill Livingstone, Edinburgh.

Chaitow, L. (1976). *The acupuncture treatment of pain.* Thorsons, Wellingborough.

Travell, J. G. and Simons, D. G. (1983). *Myofascial pain and dysfunction: the trigger point manual.* Williams and Wilcox, Baltimore.

7 Acute pain

'Acute' in medicine means of short duration and coming to a crisis. This applies to the initial pain of an incision, a fracture or a burn. It also applies to the pain of trigeminal neuralgia, the initial overwhelming onset of acute back pain, and even some migraine headaches. There has been a recent surge of interest in the important topic of pain following surgery. This follows publication of a report by the Royal Colleges of Anaesthetists and Surgeons demonstrating that pain after surgery was very poorly managed and that simple measures would relieve a lot of unnecessary suffering.

In this chapter we look at the issue of pain of short duration as a whole. Concentrating on postoperative pain would leave a large area of suffering unconsidered. A further point is that all the factors that arise from the IASP definition of pain—'an unpleasant emotional and physical experience associated with actual or potential tissue damage or described in terms of such damage'—are there in both acute and chronic pain. The pain experienced by a child having an injection or by a footballer who breaks his ankle is no less nor more than that of post-herpetic neuralgia. It is different and shorter, but it is pain.

The nature of acute pain

Acute pain differs from chronic pain in that everyone expects it to resolve and in that the sufferer can understand it. It does however generate similar suffering and anxieties. There is the anxiety of being moved and being examined, and the ignorance of the expected duration of the pain and the effect that the disease or injury may have on the sufferer's future. Acute pain is frequently unrecognized as a problem that needs treatment.

Its severity is often underestimated and, because of ignorance of the effective doses of analgesic drugs and an overestimation of the problems that might arise from their use, attempts to treat it are often inadequate. In these respects it resembles chronic pain. It was extraordinary that, 140 years after the discovery of anaesthesia and the birth of modern surgery, the Royal Colleges had to point out to both anaesthetists and surgeons that they were not treating postoperative pain effectively.

One reason why analgesia is sometimes denied is a fear that it might interfere with diagnosis, by removing the physical sign of tenderness to palpation. However, a recent study has shown that good analgesia does not eliminate tenderness. One would not expect it to; cancer pain is well controlled by opiate analgesia unless a physical stimulus, such as movement of a fracture, or pressure over the site of inflammation generates a 'new' pain stimulus. This incident pain can only be controlled by nerve blockade with a local anaesthetic or the administration of enough opiate to produce unconsciousness. It is time to end the view that patients who have not yet been diagnosed by someone senior should be denied effective analgesia. It has already resulted in a vast amount of unnecessary suffering.

Causes of acute pain

Acute pain is the pain of tissue damage, which can be a result of distortion. High-threshold mechanoceptors are specialized sensory nerve endings which signal to the CNS when tissue deformation might be sufficient to cause damage. They are present in most of the tissues in the body.

The normal response to a tissue injury is inflammation, which leads to healing. The products of inflammation are detected by nociceptor endings and signalled as pain to the CNS. Where tissue damage is extensive, venous drainage may be affected and oedema may develop, distorting tissue and stimulating high-threshold mechanoceptors, which will also signal pain. Tissue oxygen demand is increased by the process of healing, but if the supply of oxygenated blood is reduced by the wound or surgical intervention, this will cause ischaemic pain. Quick, careful surgery, gentleness, the use of position to minimize swelling, and the realization that tight sutures and dressings may cause ischaemic pain help minimize the pain of injury.

Factors affecting acute pain

One of the reasons that acute pain is undertreated and misunderstood is that we instinctively believe we know how much something should hurt.

Many things affect the intensity of pain (see Chapter 3). Only the person who has a pain knows how severe it is. One person with a Pott's fracture will grin and try to hobble away on it; another will writhe in agony.

Contribution of emotional factors

Among the most famous of all pain studies was that of Beecher (1946) who looked at the pain experienced by American soldiers wounded during the second world war on the Anzio beachhead under intense enemy fire. More than half suffered little pain at the time of their injury. Beecher speculated that this might have been because the fact of their injury would result in a release from the horror and terror of their situation. It might also have been the result of the intense excitement and distraction that resulted from having to attack the beach under enemy fire. It vividly demonstrates the effect of psychological factors on the perception of acute pain. This is an extreme example which we cannot reproduce, however by the use of explanation, reassurance, and kindness we can make use of psychological measures to minimize acute pain.

Appropriate drugs in different situations

Many things can be done to lessen and alleviate pain without the use of drugs. Drugs that relieve pain may themselves cause other problems which may be difficult to handle or even lethal. A drug that can be managed easily and safely in a hospital ward or an operating theatre may be much more difficult to control and dangerous in other circumstances. The approaches used by a medical officer on an expedition are very different from those used in an accident and emergency department, or recommended for minor accidents in the home.

Away from civilization

Travelling with opioid drugs can cause problems. Countries in which drugs of addiction can be bought in the street often have draconian controls over the import and use of these drugs for medicinal purposes. If you are planning to travel with opioid drugs, it is essential to inform the authorities in the country that you are leaving that you intend to take them with you, and to confirm with the country that you are going to that it is permissible to import them for medicinal use.

Partial agonists and NSAIDs arouse less suspicion, but it is still best to check. Morphine is the most useful drug to carry (see p. 47 for details). It can be given by mouth if there is no one with the skills to give it parenterally, and enough morphine to relieve a great deal of pain takes up little space.

There is no point in taking other opioid analgesics to faraway places. In the rare circumstances in which morphine might make matters worse, for example in renal or gall bladder colic, an NSAID which can be given intravenously gives consistent relief. Ketorolac is currently the best of these available, but if this is impracticable diclofenac by suppository works well. A 30 mg dose of ketorolac is as potent as 10 mg of morphine. It is slower in onset than morphine, and like other drugs in its class there is a plateau in its dose–response relationship, so in some circumstances it will not produce satisfactory pain relief.

This problem of a plateau in effect also applies to the partial opioid agonists, making these drugs less valuable than morphine, however they may be the only powerful analgesics that can be taken. Buprenorphine is the most powerful of the partial agonists. As it is absorbed through the buccal mucosa, it provides analgesia of rapid onset, and will work even if the gastrointestinal tract is not functioning. It is long acting, one dose being sufficient for six hours. It is metabolized in the liver to a considerable extent, so is not very effective if swallowed. In about a third of people it causes severe nausea and, as the drug is so long acting, this can be extremely distressing. It has become one of the abused drugs and is now subject to many of the same controls as morphine.

Pentazocine is not as powerful as buprenorphine, and can cause a most unpleasant dysphoria, which would be distressing a long way from civilization. Nalbuphine is not so commonly used. Although it is not as powerful as buprenorphine, it seems to have few problems and might be worth taking on an expedition.

Local anaesthetics can be useful for peripheral injuries. Three are in common use in the UK—prilocaine, lignocaine, and bupivacaine. Prilocaine has half the toxicity of lignocaine and has a similar time of onset of action. It has the disadvantage of causing methaemoglobinaemia, but when it is used in clinical doses this is rarely significant. Lignocaine and prilocaine are more rapid in onset than buprenorphine which is the longest lasting.

Local anaesthetics can be toxic when absorbed systemically, so it is important to be aware of the maximum recommended doses and of how much you are giving, in milligrams. The maximum recommended dose of prilocaine is 8 mg per kg, or 480 mg for a medium-sized adult. For lignocaine, it is 4 mg per kg, or 240 mg for a medium-sized adult, if given in a plain solution. If they are given mixed with adrenalin to delay absorption, the dose is doubled. A 1 per cent solution will provide good pain relief if infiltrated around a wound into damaged tissue or into a fracture. For most adults the maximum volume that should be used is about 50 ml of prilocaine plain or 100 ml of prilocaine with adrenalin (25 ml of ligno-caine plain or 50 ml with adrenalin). If the drug is given intravenously or onto a mucous membrane through which it may be rapidly absorbed the toxicity becomes much greater. These routes are therefore not recom-mended for use if resuscitation facilities and skills are not immediately available.

It is beyond the scope of this book to describe nerve blocks. However, even in difficult circumstances, it is possible to perform axillary brachial plexus blocks and inject local anaesthetic into the epidural space through the sacral hiatus, a caudal block. These blocks anaesthetize the upper limb and lower part of the lower limbs, respectively. A femoral nerve block gives useful pain relief for the upper part of the lower limb. If you might be expected to provide surgical anaesthesia away from civilization it would be useful to learn these blocks from an expert before going.

In the street and at home

Providing relief for acute pain in the street and in the home can make a considerable difference to an injured or sick person's suffering, but it often takes a low priority. If oral medication is all that is available, it is better than nothing as it will provide effective analgesia after a delay. Oral morphine sulphate tablets work in half an hour, and powerful NSAIDs such as ibuprofen and diclofenac, nearly as quickly.

If the pain is great morphine can be given intravenously, and this is a better route than intramuscular injection. Hypovolaemic patients absorb the drug from intramuscular sites slowly, until the circulation improves. And even when the peripheral circulation is good, absorption from intra-muscular injection is very variable.

Morphine takes effect about five minutes after an intravenous injection. The best and safest way to use it is to give small increments of 2 mg at intervals of five minutes until pain has become tolerable. An overdose of morphine will of course result in respiratory depression, but this is signi-ficant only at much greater doses than are needed for good pain relief.

Inhalational analgesia using 50 per cent nitrous oxide in oxygen works well in the street or the home. Ambulances now carry entonox. It takes two minutes of inhalation for the nitrous oxide to replace the nitrogen in the body and to reach the best possible level of analgesia.

Where disease is generating severe pain there is no reason not to provide rapid intense relief by giving opioid intravenously. The safest way to give morphine in this situation is to give small increments, wait for any effect, and then repeat. The pain itself tends to counteract the drowsiness and respiratory depression that morphine causes. However, when this technique is used, the morphine antidote naloxone should be available, and the person administering it should know how to resuscitate. When naloxone is used to counteract an overdose of morphine, it is important to remember that if large doses are given rapidly all the effects of morphine, including pain relief, will be lost. Further doses of morphine will be in-effective for up to an hour. Naloxone, like morphine, should be given in small incremental doses.

Intramuscular or intravenous doses of NSAIDs may be safer in these circumstances. They take longer to take effect than morphine and they are not totally safe. However, they do not cause respiratory depression. If there is a possibility that the patient is seeking an opioid because of addiction, or for pleasure, then an NSAID will relieve pain while not causing other problems.

These drugs may cause renal failure in patients with diminished renal function, or who are dehydrated, and they may cause haemorrhage in patients with a history of peptic ulceration or indigestion, even if not taken by mouth. Ketorolac is the only preparation that can currently be given intravenously, and a dose of 10 mg will produce good analgesia in an adult in about 30 minutes. Diclofenac is quite powerful and can be given intramuscularly or by suppository.

Patients who have severe pain may be very distressed and anxious, and this may contribute to their pain. A rapidly acting benzodiazepine such as midazolam given intravenously, or an oral dose of a tricyclic antidepress-ant such as amitriptyline, may relieve an acute pain that seems to be getting out of control despite liberal use of analgesics.

Analgesics to keep at home

People ask advice on the most suitable pain control measures for use by the unqualified. Many people with no knowledge of pharmacology have no idea of the dangers that are associated with taking simple, readily available drugs like aspirin and paracetamol. It might be better and safer to tolerate some pain from a headache or sprain which is not interfering with enjoyment of life than to assume that all pain should be relieved by medication.

The safest pain relief methods available are stimulation methods and these can be unexpectedly effective. A bag of frozen peas over a sprain or a stiff neck, a well wrapped hot water bottle over an aching stomach, firm finger pressure over a myofascial trigger point in the neck or back, or oil of wintergreen rubbed into an area of muscle stiffness are all completely safe and often very effective.

Paracetamol is the safest analgesic, but it is toxic in overdose. This is not widely known, and overdoses intended as a gesture too often become suicide in reality. Paracetamol is combined with opioids in many widely used preparations (see Chapter 5), and it is the paracetamol that determines the maximum dose rather than the more powerful and effective opioid (Table 7.1). A recent survey found that many doctors were not aware of the contents of these preparations or the potential toxicity of the paracetamol.

Table 7.1 Combined preparations containing paracetamol

Preparation	Opioid content (normal dose of opioid alone in brackets)	Paracetamol content	Dosage interval for two tablets (max. 4 g paracetamol per day)
Co-proxamol	Dextropoxyphene 32.5 mg (60 mg)	325 mg	4 hours
Co-codamol	Codeine 8 mg or 10 mg (60 mg, max. 200 mg/day)	500 mg	6 hours
Co-dydramol	Codeine 8 mg (10 mg)	500 mg	6 hours

The tablets which combine paracetamol with an opioid are neither better nor safer than the opioid on its own. Indeed the amounts of opioid in the mixtures are often little different from the unmixed preparation. The *British National Formulary* recommends that these combinations should not be used, but this sensible piece of pharmacological advice is widely disregarded. It would be better to prescribe the two components separately, but many people could not cope with the demands of taking two drugs, one four hourly and another six hourly.

Drugs with a short duration of action such as pethidine and dextromoramide have no place in this area. They are prescribed at intervals longer than their duration of action. This would produce a short period of pain relief followed by a long interval, in pain, before the next dose and freedom from pain—the perfect recipe for generating dependence.

If intense analgesia is needed through drugs taken at home then morphine is probably the best drug. The only exception is pain caused by smooth muscle spasm, as morphine increases the tone of smooth muscle. Immediate pain relief should be provided by a rapidly acting preparation such as Sevredol and maintained by slow-release morphine, which only takes effect two and a half hours after the dose is taken.

Where there is smooth muscle spasm, for example in renal colic or gall bladder colic, then ketorolac given intravenously or intramuscularly, or diclofenac given intramuscularly or by suppository is best. But it is important to remember the dangers associated with all NSAIDs when using these drugs.

In hospital

Once someone in pain has reached hospital all methods of pain relief become available, and there are few if any reasons why they should remain in pain. The cause of pain and its proper management should be assessed as soon after arrival as possible.

Postoperative pain should be assessed regularly and analgesia given whenever needed. This is acknowledged by all those who wish to improve pain management. There is no reason not to extend this doctrine to all patients in hospital, from the moment of their arrival. The severity of pain will change as the patient becomes more or less anxious, as a result of physical examination and X-ray investigations. There is therefore a case for keeping pain charts for all patients if they have been admitted with, or might develop, pain (see Chapter 4).

Simple methods are best—where oral medication will do the job efficiently, it is better than parenteral. Severe pain needs intravenous opioid, mild pain an NSAID. Inhalational analgesia with nitrous oxide–oxygen mixture (entonox) will provide instant rapid relief, but must be inhaled for at least two minutes to be effective.

The measures to relieve pain are all rapidly available in hospital, as are the skills to use them; what is sometimes missing is the recognition that pain exists, and the will to do something about it and to take advice when it persists in spite of attempts to relieve it.

Complications and hazards

Everything has its price and the benefit from pain relief must be set against the price paid in terms of side-effects. It is perfectly normal for human beings not to wish to receive a treatment, and to prefer to experience some pain rather than take an analgesic.

Inhalational analgesia Entonox is the only inhalational analgesic in common use. It is also one of the safest. However, if air is trapped in a body cavity, for example a pneumothorax, the nitrous oxide will enter that cavity more rapidly than the nitrogen in the air can leave, so increasing either the volume or the pressure in the space.

If nitrous oxide is inhaled for more than 48 hours, it will interfere with folic acid metabolism causing a megaloblastic anaemia.

Nitrous oxide–oxygen mixtures strongly support combustion, so there is a danger of conflagration or explosion if it is used in the presence of a combustible material and a source of ignition.

If the temperature of an entonox cylinder falls below 4°C the nitrous oxide and oxygen separate and the mixture will not reform until the cylinder has been rewarmed and inverted several times. If this is not done, the patient will get first pure oxygen and no pain relief, and then pure nitrous oxide which will be quickly lethal.

Mild analgesics and NSAIDs   All mild analgesics and NSAIDs may be toxic to both the liver and kidney if the function of these organs is already impaired. Paracetamol is the safest of these drugs, but if taken in overdose its metabolites cannot be safely conjugated in the liver and cause fatal liver failure.

Aspirin and all the other drugs in this group interfere with the synthesis of prostaglandin. This reduces the protective barrier on the gastric wall, leading to erosion, ulceration, and bleeding. They also interfere with the production of thromboxane, and decrease the adhesiveness of platelets, so making any haemorrhage more severe. People may be hypersensitive to all these drugs and may have an anaphylactic response to them.

It is generally believed that these drugs should be the analgesics of first choice because they are less powerful, and the analgesia is due to their anti-inflammatory effect and therefore partially therapeutic. It is true that they do not cause dependence or drowsiness but they are not safer—they can be lethal as can any other type of analgesic.

Opioids   All opioids exert their analgesic effects through an interaction with the mu receptor on nociceptor neurons. They also interact with other mu receptors, and so cause nausea and anorexia, respiratory depression leading to respiratory arrest, spasm of smooth muscle causing mydriasis, spasm of intestinal muscle causing constipation, and drowsiness. There is no evidence that analgesic doses of any one produces lesser side-effects than analgesic doses of any other. Drugs that have the reputation for inducing less drowsiness, or less respiratory depression, are just less potent.

There are differences, however. Pethidine relaxes some smooth muscle and produces better pain relief in colic pains. Pethidine and dextropoxyphene cause convulsions in overdose. Codeine and dihydrocodeine cause headache. They may be more powerful cough suppressants than equianalgesic doses of morphine.

Local anaesthetic Local anaesthetic causes convulsions and cardiac arrest in overdose. The highest blood levels and thus the greatest potential toxicity occur when they are given intravenously, but rapid rises in blood level also happen when they are sprayed onto mucous membranes or injected into inflamed tissue.

Hypovolaemia and head injury

A patient who has lost blood will react to analgesics differently from other patients. Tissue perfusion is reduced, so drugs given intramuscularly or subcutaneously will be absorbed more slowly, if at all. And drugs given intravenously will be diluted by a smaller volume of blood before reaching their target, so will be at higher concentration. All this means that patients who have lost enough blood to cause a tachycardia, a fall in blood pressure, pallor, or all three should be given analgesic, but in small incremental intravenous doses. The intramuscular route is particularly dangerous, because further doses may be given when the first appears to be ineffective. When the circulation is restored by transfusion, the drug in its intramuscular depot is absorbed and a relative overdose can result.

Head injury can cause bleeding in the cranial cavity leading to an increase in intracranial pressure as the blood cannot escape from the enclosed space of the skull. The pressure rises further if the level of carbon dioxide in arterial blood increases as a result of respiratory depression, because the blood flow to the brain increases, tending to increase its volume. Opioid drugs depress respiration so they should not be used if there is any question that there might be an intracranial bleed.

Patients who have had a head injury are monitored for signs of deterioration, which may indicate a bleed, including increasing drowsiness and a change in the size of the pupils. As opioids affect both of these indicators, they interfere with monitoring—another reason why they should not be used in head injury.

NSAIDs should not be used if there is any risk that reducing blood coagulability will cause further haemorrhage. Regional analgesia may be the only way to produce pain relief from a peripheral injury.

The role of nerve blocks

Local anaesthetic techniques seem superficially to be a safe and effective way of producing pain relief, but they have dangers and should be used with caution. In many circumstances only anaesthetists who have had extensive training will be able to use local anaesthetic techniques to provide pain relief. However, some techniques can be used by nonspecialists. For example, a fracture haematoma can be infiltrated to produce enough analgesia for manipulation or the application of a splint. Strict asepsis is important, as the danger from an infection is very great. When large volumes of local anaesthetic are injected there is always the possibility of systemic toxicity developing suddenly; it is a wise precaution to cannulate a vein first.

Other local anaesthetic techniques for pain relief have been described in the section on pain relief away from civilization (p. 00). If you use local anaesthetic drugs always be aware of their toxicity. They produce first convulsions, then cardiac arrest. Do not use large amounts of local anaesthetic unless there are resuscitation facilities and people available who can use them quickly and efficiently.

Resuscitation facilities

All doctors and nurses should be competent at resuscitation. When there is no one competent to resuscitate, sophisticated pain relief techniques should not be used. The principal dangers are sudden delayed respiratory depression and hypotension. There must be a nearby supply of the morphine antidote naloxone, and an infusion running so that fluid can be given rapidly if necessary. A method for giving artificial ventilation and someone who can use it must also be close at hand.

Opioid infusions, epidural infusions and patient-controlled analgesia

The only way to use these techniques safely and effectively is to watch the patient closely, to keep a regular pain chart and to be prepared to modify the amount of analgesic being delivered frequently.

The aim of an opioid infusion is to produce a constant analgesic level of opioid in the blood. It is probably the least effective of these analgesic techniques, as it has little effect on the incident pain that movement causes.

Patient-controlled analgesia In patient-controlled analgesia (PCA) a syringe pump delivers a preset dose of analgesic with a preset minimum interval between doses. Patients press a button to deliver the next dose. If the machine has been set up with too small a dose of analgesic and too long a 'lock-out' interval between doses, patients can find themselves trapped and unable to get effective pain relief. It is therefore vital that pain assessment is done thoroughly and frequently. If the analgesia is inadequate, the dose should be increased; if the analgesia is wearing off before the next dose can be delivered, the lock-out interval should be shortened. Most people will need about 5 mg of intravenous morphine for effective analgesia. They should be able to get this amount in 20 minutes.

It should be impossible for a patient to overdose using PCA, unless the single dose is set too high; after all, patients who have had more than enough morphine fall asleep and so will not push the button on their PCA. However, if they are woken and asked if they are in pain, the awakening causes incident pain. The patient may then press the PCA button to get more morphine, which can cause respiratory depression. These devices work best when both the patients and staff understand how to use them and are enthusiastic about them. Patients should be given instructions before having their operations.

Epidural infusions Morphine works by blocking the reception of pain impulses as they arrive at the dorsal horn of the spinal cord. When it is given by intramuscular or intravenous injection the proportion of the total dose that gets to this site is very small. The rest is distributed to other parts of the body, and causes the unwanted sedation, nausea, respiratory depression, and constipation. If morphine can be introduced near to the cord, very small doses will produce intense analgesia. Morphine is much more soluble in water than in fat, so when it gets into the cerebrospinal fluid (CSF) it stays there for a long time, and does not dissolve in the fatty material of which the spinal cord is made. If it is put into the epidural space it does not dissolve in the epidural fat but diffuses across the dura into the CSF. It is therefore very effective given by this route. The problem is that it may eventually diffuse up to the brain and bathe the respiratory centre in morphine, producing a delayed and intense respiratory depression.

When fat-soluble analgesics such as pethidine, fentanyl, and methadone are given epidurally they dissolve in the epidural fat and are absorbed into the circulation. What does diffuse across the dura does not remain in the CSF bathing the dorsal horn neurones, but dissolves in the cord and is cleared by the circulation. These drugs are therefore little more effective given this way than when they are given intravenously. Diamorphine is more fat-soluble than morphine, but is rapidly metabolized to morphine and monoacetyl morphine. Because it is more fat soluble, less free morphine gets into the CSF than when morphine itself is given epidurally. This makes it safer than morphine, but still effective, because enough morphine remains in the CSF.

Local anaesthetic injected epidurally will block pain and other transmission. However, concentrations that produce good pain relief cause an uncomfortable numbness, and even some motor block. Above the second lumbar dermatome it will also block some of the sympathetic outflow and may cause hypotension.

A mixture of local anaesthetic and morphine is much more effective than either alone. We use 5 mg of diamorphine in 60 ml of 0.167 per cent bupivacaine for epidural infusion over 12 hours or more. These small amounts are extremely effective.

The dangers of epidural infusions are delayed respiratory depression and hypotension. They will not be effective if the solution does not get onto the nerve roots supplying the wound. All this means that patients given epidural infusions need frequent monitoring of blood pressure, respiratory rate, and of course pain. If part of the wound is painful then the rate of infusion should be increased. If respiratory depression starts then the patient should be given respiratory support if needed, and naloxone. If the blood pressure falls remember that patients can bleed after surgery, and have myocardial infarctions, so check for all possible causes, rather than assuming it is due to the epidural. Give crystalloid fluid fast, and a small dose of vasopressor such as ephedrine or vasoxamine if you are sure that the cause of the blood pressure fall is the epidural infusion.

Management of postoperative pain

First look at what is safely possible. All staff must be trained in all techniques that are being used, otherwise they can be both ineffective and dangerous. All patients who have surgery should have pain and nausea monitored, as well as the other vital signs. When PCA or epidural infusions are not feasible, intramuscular morphine given liberally when needed can give postoperative pain relief as good as that provided by any other technique, but the doctors prescribing it must understand about pain perception, and the nurses who have the responsibility for delivering it must understand how to use morphine effectively, and be trusted by the doctors.

The patient must also understand what techniques are available for dealing with postoperative pain and make an informed choice about which is to be used. Then all those who have a responsibility to provide pain relief after surgery must be taught about the value, management, and dangers of the analgesic techniques that are available. When a specific postoperative analgesia service is running, its value and safety depend entirely on effective supervision.

Even when simple techniques are chosen it is worth infiltrating the wound with local anaesthetic, and giving an NSAID (unless it might cause complications) and an opiate. Enthusiasm and education are the keys to the relief of pain after surgery.

References

Beecher, H. K. (1946). Pain in men wounded in battle. *Annals of Surgery*, 123, 96.
Merskey, H. (1986). Classification of chronic pain. Description of chronic pain syndromes and definitions of pain terms. *Pain* (Suppl.), 3, S1–S225.

8 Pain in cancer

The relief of the physical, mental, and social symptoms of disease in the dying has become the basis of palliative care. Among the most distressing of these symptoms is pain associated with malignant disease. Relieving it is not curative treatment and does not alter the disease process, and yet it is not necessarily 'terminal care'. Relief of distressing symptoms should begin whenever they arise and not be reserved for the terminal stages. Although pain is often thought to be the main symptom in cancer, and will be the main consideration in this chapter, palliative care should aim to ameliorate all the distressing symptoms in a patient with malignant disease.

Pain is certainly a common symptom of cancer, affecting about 70 per cent of patients. It has been suggested that at least 50 per cent of patients undergoing treatment for cancer continue to suffer pain and, although the management of pain has improved tremendously in recent years, it is still frequently neglected in favour of disease management. However, the growth of hospices and their philosophy have given symptom management a higher profile and—together with the growth of palliative care teams in hospitals and in the community—have raised awareness of the importance of this aspect of patient care.

Pain in a patient with cancer may be a direct result of the cancer but it may also be unrelated—a feature, perhaps, of long-standing musculoskeletal disease. Pain may arise because of the debilitating effects of the disease, or even as a result of treatment. Surgery and radiotherapy may produce painful secondary effects. Many patients with cancer have several pains arising from different sources or pathologies, and it is important to assess the likely cause of each in order to apply the most appropriate treatment. The pains of visceral distension, nerve compression, bone erosion, and intestinal obstruction need different therapeutic approaches. It is also essential to consider whether pain is being aggravated by mental pain and anguish at the prospect of impending decline, or by other distressing but non-painful conditions.

Pain associated with cancer is chronic in that it is ongoing, generally has no natural tendency to resolve, and is often accompanied by many of the psychological features of chronic pain. There may also be irreversible damage to nervous tissue which is often a feature of other chronic pain syndromes. However, cancer pain is also acute in that much of it results from stimulation of nociceptors. It is a continuing and progressive disease process that produces pain by tissue damage, distortion, and inflammation.

Goals in pain management

It is important to determine realistic aims in the management of pain, and these should where possible be discussed with the patient. It may not be possible to relieve all pain associated with cancer, but it is nearly always possible to provide some relief from distressing symptoms and improve the quality of life. Most patients would agree that to obtain a reasonable night's rest should be the first goal. Pain which disturbs sleep is perhaps most difficult for the patient to cope with. The next aim is usually to relieve pain at rest during daytime. The last—and often the most difficult to achieve—is pain-free activity. There may have to be some compromise between achieving complete freedom from pain on movement, and the unacceptable side-effects from pain-relieving drugs or other treatments. Many patients will accept this compromise provided that they have adequate reassurance and support.

After establishing the aims of pain management, it is helpful to identify likely origins of the pain. This will help to determine the most effective way of treating it. Pain arising in viscera, and deep, aching pain are often best managed with opioid drugs. Their psychogenic effects may also have an important benefit. Pain which arises in the musculoskeletal system, especially if there is an element of inflammation, may be relieved by the use of a non-steroidal anti-inflammatory drug (NSAID), either alone or combined with an opioid.

Compression or destruction of nervous tissue may result in sharp shooting pains. Alternatively it may cause a burning type of pain, which is often associated with dysaesthesia and allodynia, when normal touch stimuli may produce an unpleasant painful sensation. These pains may respond better to an anticonvulsant drug or a tricyclic antidepressant than to an opioid or NSAID. Neurogenic pain and pain arising in bone may be relatively unresponsive to opioids and it is important to consider other types of drugs and alternative therapies in their management.

Analgesic drugs

Analgesics are usually the first choice for pain control in malignant disease. Invasive and destructive procedures were popular in the past, but are now generally a second choice. Analgesic drugs can be titrated against the pain and adjusted in the light of benefits and side-effects. They are reversible and generally involve the patient to some extent in symptom control, rather than their being the passive recipient of technical procedures. This may have some psychological benefits. In countries where potent analgesics are not freely prescribable, destructive procedures are more often necessary.

It is only by sensitive assessment of both beneficial and unwanted effects by well-trained and dedicated nursing staff that the optimum use of analgesics can be obtained. Too frequently medical staff prescribe set 'formulary' doses of drugs without adequate follow-up, resulting in ineffective treatment or intolerable side-effects. Rapid reassessment allows determination of the optimum analgesic regimen.

There are no set doses for the strong opioid drugs. The correct dose is that which provides maximum analgesia with minimum side-effects. This means that there is a wide scope for titrating dose against response. The weaker opioids tend to have a low analgesic ceiling, so that increasing the dose does not increase analgesia but produces unacceptable side-effects. Other analgesics such as paracetamol or anti-inflammatory drugs have dose-related toxic effects which restrict the dose range and hence flexibility of use. Strong opioid analgesics offer a much greater flexibility in dose, even when used in low doses.

Administration of analgesic drugs should be planned to produce a constant effect, rather than taken 'when necessary'. If a drug with a relatively short period of action is administered too infrequently, the fluctuating levels of analgesia result in poor pain control. The repeated rises in plasma levels alternating with withdrawal of effect are distressing to the patient. Long-lasting pain requires long-lasting analgesia. Drugs should be given 'by the clock' at regular intervals depending on the period of activity of the drug. It is generally preferable to select a longer-acting drug for maintenance. This may be best provided by a sustained-release preparation such as MST Continus tablets, or by a long-acting opioid such as methadone. However, a shorter-acting preparation may be required for initial assessment of the appropriate dose.

The pain which the patient experiences, rather than the stage of the disease, should determine the type of analgesic prescribed. Opioid drugs are frequently kept from patients until the late stages of the disease in the erroneous belief that starting potent analgesics too early means there will be nothing effective left later, because the patient will have become tolerant to the analgesic. There is also often some reluctance to start giving regular strong opioids to a patient who is ambulant and trying to continue some form of normal life. It is certainly true that many patients with cancer only have pain which is easily managed with simple analgesics or weak opioids, but if these are inadequate then there is no logical reason not to prescribe morphine or similar analgesics, whatever the life expectancy.

The only real requirement is that the patient has a pain which is responsive to opioid analgesics. Many patients can be managed on a constant dose of morphine for long periods if it is high enough to achieve pain control. There may be some gradual development of tolerance, but this usually reaches a plateau at about three months and demands for increasing dose are more likely to represent a progression of the disease than the further development of tolerance. Usually the patient will only request a higher dose if the pain is inadequately controlled. Tolerance to side-effects such as drowsiness and nausea usually develops over the first few days or weeks (see p. 62). Once a stabilized effective dose has been reached, the use of opioid drugs may permit a greater return to normal life than if pain is inadequately controlled by weaker analgesics.

Many patients are concerned that they may become addicted to opioid drugs. This fear is often confirmed by their doctor's concern and reluctance to prescribe such drugs until the final days. It is important to reassure patients that addiction has little real meaning when the drugs are being properly used for pain control. When pain is controlled with constant levels of analgesic drug with few peaks and troughs in plasma levels, there is unlikely to be any drug-seeking behaviour, certainly not similar to that in people who consume drugs for a psychogenic effect. If pain is later relieved by some other means, such as a therapeutic nerve block, patients can usually be weaned off their opioid drugs fairly easily and rapidly. Some physical dependence may develop, but this is not a problem if therapy is to be continued, and it is easily dealt with, if necessary, by gradual reduction in dose if opioids are no longer required. This is not 'addiction'.

The analgesic staircase

Analgesic drugs can be considered as steps on a staircase. The first step includes the simple non-opioid analgesics and the NSAIDs. If these are insufficient then the prescriber should move onto the second step, which includes the weak opioids. Finally, at the top of the staircase are the strong opioid analgesics.

The conventional view has been that a patient should only move up the staircase when the weaker drugs have been ineffective. This concept has value in emphasizing that there is no point in substituting another drug from the same potency group for one that has been found to be ineffective. However, it overlooks the point that drugs considered to be of similar potency may have different modes of action (for example paracetamol and an NSAID) and therefore they may be more effective when used together, or with a drug from a different step, than when used alone.

Another limitation of the staircase concept is that patients with severe pain may spend an unnecessary amount of time on the lower steps when they should receive a potent analgesic at an early stage. It could also be argued that a small dose of a potent drug such as morphine is no less safe than a large dose of codeine. It may be more effective, with fewer side-effects, and increasing the dose still has some benefit if the level of pain increases.

Overall, the best advice is to assess the level and type of pain which the patient reports. If it is relatively mild then it may be well controlled with a simple analgesic. If pain is severe then it is justifiable to use potent analgesics at the earliest stage.

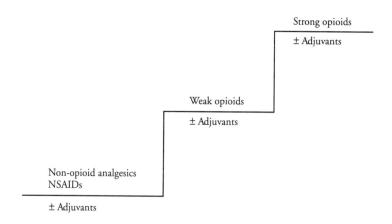

Fig. 8.1 The analgesic staircase.

Opioid-resistant pain

Although it is occasionally necessary to use very high doses of opioid to control pain in patients with cancer, most can be successfully managed with relatively low doses. However, it is important to recognize when pain is not responsive, or is only partially responsive, to opioids. This is the case for pain arising from compressed or damaged nervous tissue, and pain from bone erosions and fractures which may only be apparent on movement. No dose of morphine will satisfactorily control the pain resulting from weight bearing on a fractured bone. For these pains, additional or alternative drugs or physical means of relieving pain will be needed.

Starting opioid therapy

Good pain management requires close monitoring of the effects of analgesic administration and patients in severe pain initially need frequent supervision.

It is often easiest to start with regular four-hourly morphine elixir. The starting dose will depend on several factors, such as renal and hepatic function, and the age and general degree of debility of the patient. Most patients who are not already on some form of opioid start on a dose of around 5–10 mg four hourly. For patients who have already had a poor response to opioid analgesics, the previous dose should be converted to an equivalent dose of morphine and then increased by 50 per cent. The dose can then be titrated against the patient's pain by increasing the dose once or twice a day in increments of 30–50 per cent.

There is no standard dose for morphine and there is huge variation in the dose required from one individual to another. Some patients will require several hundred milligrams, although most will be satisfactorily managed on less than 200 mg per day. The correct dose is that which most effectively controls the pain with tolerable side-effects. Table 8.1 gives equivalent doses of some opioid drugs.

Table 8.1 Approximate equivalents to oral morphine 10 mg, 4 hourly

Diamorphine (oral)	10 mg	4 hourly
Methadone (oral)	10 mg	6–8 hourly
Controlled-release morphine tablets (MST)	30 mg	12 hourly
Phenazocine (sublingual)	5 mg	6–8 hourly
Oxycodone (suppository)	30 mg	8 hourly
Buprenorphine (sublingual)	0.6 mg	6 hourly

Managing pain in out-patients should be arranged in close cooperation with the community nursing services. It may not be easy for the patient to titrate the dose against the pain regularly and effectively without adequate supervision and advice at home. Many patients can adjust their dose themselves provided that clear guidelines are given. If good home support is not possible, or if the pain is severe, it may occasionally be best to admit the patient to a hospital or hospice for a short period to stabilize analgesic therapy.

As soon as the dose of morphine needed to provide a stable level of analgesia is known, the patient should be started on a controlled-release form. Morphine elixir can be converted milligram for milligram to controlled-release tablets: the total daily dose of elixir can be divided into two and administered as two 12-hourly doses. This provides a constant level of analgesia and is more convenient for the patient and their attendants. Occasionally it is necessary to increase the frequency of administration to eight hourly, but it is generally better to increase the 12-hourly dose than increase the frequency. This formulation of morphine is not suitable for more frequent administration and should certainly never be given on an 'as required' basis.

If there is an urgent need to control severe pain, then it may be necessary to administer morphine in incremental doses intravenously. If satisfactory analgesia can be obtained in this way, conversion to an oral preparation can be made when the patient can take oral medication. The intravenous dose should be multiplied by three to give an equivalent four-hourly oral dose, to take into account the lower bioavailability of oral morphine.

Maintaining analgesia during the night is especially important and may present a problem when pain is controlled during the daytime with a shorter-acting preparation, such as morphine sulphate elixir. This can usually be managed by doubling the dose taken in the late evening and then omitting the dose which would be due four hours later, so eliminating the need to wake the patient for medication. An alternative is to use a morphine or oxycodone suppository at night. This will provide good drug delivery during sleep, and oxycodone will generally last throughout the night.

Managing side-effects

Patients may suffer nausea when starting opioid therapy and it is usually helpful to prescribe an antiemetic routinely at this stage. As tolerance to the emetic effect often develops within a few weeks, it may become unnecessary to continue antiemetic medication. Continuing nausea may result more from the disease process than from the opioid drugs. Nausea associated with opioid medication usually responds to drugs such as prochlorperazine or domperidone. If nausea makes oral administration of drugs difficult initially, they can be given in the form of a suppository. If nausea persists, then haloperidol 0.5–5 mg twice daily is usually effective.

Patients may also experience sedation on starting opioid therapy. This may be partly due to exhaustion caused by unrelieved pain. After a few nights of improved sleep, the sedative effect becomes less noticeable. However, the analgesic drugs do have a direct sedative effect, which usually decreases over a few days as tolerance develops. If unacceptable sleepiness continues it may be necessary to reduce the dose slightly and then increase it again as tolerance to sedation develops.

Constipation is an almost invariable accompaniment to opioid therapy. A bowel stimulant and faecal softener (such as the combination drugs co-danthramer or co-danthrusate) should be prescribed routinely, at least in the early stages of opioid use. It may be possible to use smaller and less frequent doses later. It is important not to administer such stimulant

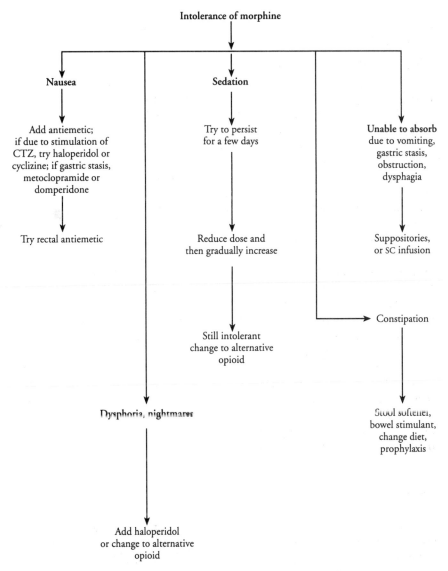

Fig. 8.2 Actions to take if a patient tolerates morphine poorly. CTZ, chemoreceptor trigger zone.

laxatives if there is a possibility of intestinal obstruction or if the patient complains of colicky abdominal pains. Lactulose is frequently prescribed, although it is not as effective as these other laxatives and can sometimes produce a feeling of flatulence and abdominal distension.

Figure 8.2 summarizes actions to take when a patient cannot tolerate morphine.

Choice of drug

When pain is not controlled in spite of large doses of morphine, it may be because the pain is partially or even completely opioid unresponsive (see p. 60). If pain is arising from invasion of bone or damage to nervous tissue by a tumour, or if acute pain is superimposed on chronic pain (for example by movement of a pathological fracture) other methods must be tried.

There is little to choose between morphine and diamorphine taken orally for control of pain in cancer. It is claimed that diamorphine may be more acceptable to patients, producing less nausea, but this is difficult to substantiate. However, only morphine is available in a sustained-release formulation and diamorphine is not available for medicinal use in most countries.

Morphine elixirs are often flavoured. The practice of adding chloroform water to morphine as a preservative makes it taste unpleasant and may not be essential to produce an acceptable shelf life. The addition of other drugs to morphine elixir, such as chlorpromazine, cocaine, and gin or brandy to produce a 'Brompton cocktail', is no longer considered desirable. These drugs may have unpleasant side-effects and administering them in a fixed dose ratio with morphine limits the flexibility of opioid dose. It is better to give antiemetics separately, and to use drugs without the sedative properties of chlorpromazine. Cocaine can be dysphoriant. Alcohol often has great merits in palliative care by acting as an appetite stimulant, mild relaxant, and social catalyst, but is better administered by more traditional means. Taking opioid analgesics does not preclude moderate consumption of alcoholic drinks, although patients will need to be aware of the potentially enhanced sedative effects.

Parenteral administration of opioids

The oral route is the first choice for administration of analgesics, but there are times when this becomes difficult, for example because of nausea and vomiting. Absorption may be ineffective due to gastrointestinal obstruction or stasis. Swallowing may be difficult in the later stages of disease, and ultimately impaired consciousness may preclude oral medication.

Suppositories or sublingual medication can be tried, but both of these options may be limited by factors such as diarrhoea, localized pain, and dryness of the mouth. It is also difficult to administer the large doses of opioids that may be required in the later stages by these routes.

Parenteral administration may then be necessary. Intramuscular injection is not suitable for long-term use because of its traumatic and intermittent nature. It is better to give the drugs by continuous subcutaneous infusion. Not only is this less traumatic for the patient, but also it may give better pain relief with fewer side-effects because more controlled plasma levels can be achieved. The development of small battery-operated syringe drivers has enabled this means of drug delivery to be readily available and it can even be used in ambulant patients.

Poor pain control is not necessarily an indication for use of a subcutaneous infusion, but occasionally this method can achieve good pain control in a patient whose opioid-sensitive pain has proved difficult to control by other means. It may then be possible to switch back to oral medication.

The use of a syringe driver during the final stages of illness, when the patient is unable to take oral medication, helps to control distressing symptoms in a way which minimizes trauma to the patient and distress to the relatives.

Continuous subcutaneous infusion devices need a pump that is lightweight and portable, simple to use and reliable. The simplest and most popular in the UK consists of a battery-operated syringe driver which takes a 10 ml syringe (Fig. 8.3). The driver can be programmed to deliver the contents of the syringe over a period of up to 24 hours. This is ideal as it means that a very small volume of infusion is delivered at a constant rate and can be readily absorbed. The device can be worn in a shoulder holster by ambulant patients and there is an audiovisual warning when the syringe is empty or the battery is low.

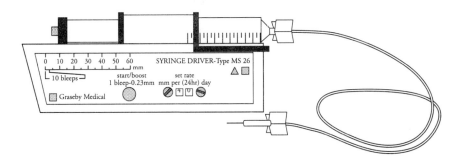

Fig. 8.3 A syringe driver for subcutaneous infusion.

The total dose of drugs to be administered by infusion over 24 hours should always be diluted to 10 ml and administered from a 10 ml syringe. If the dose of any of the drugs is to be changed, it is better to change the concentration of the drug in the syringe rather than to alter the rate of infusion. This keeps the infusate volume to a level which can be easily absorbed, and also reduces errors in setting the pump controls. Larger volumes infused over 24 hours will be uncomfortable for the patient and increase the incidence of local skin problems.

The syringe is connected to a long-tailed winged infusion needle, the tubing primed, and the needle inserted subcutaneously at an angle of approximately 45° into previously cleaned skin. The anterior chest wall is usually a comfortable and convenient site although other relatively flat and immobile areas may have to be used. The wings of the needle can be secured to the skin with a non-irritant adhesive dressing and can remain in place for long periods. Induration may develop, but it is only necessary to change the site if it becomes inflamed. Long-term use is rarely necessary, but when it is indicated there is no absolute limit to the period of use of subcutaneous infusion. Before starting the infusion it is usually necessary to administer a loading dose of analgesic and possibly antiemetic, since the slow infusion means it can take a long time to achieve effective levels of drugs.

All the drugs listed in Table 8.2 as suitable for use with subcutaneous infusion are compatible and can be mixed in the same syringe. In practice,

Table 8.2   Drugs suitable for subcutaneous infusion

Drug	Indications	Starting dose (24 hours)
Diamorphine	Pain	20 mg (if not already on opioid)
Cyclizine	Nausea, intestinal obstruction	100–150 mg
Metoclopramide	Impaired gastric emptying	30–40 mg
Haloperidol	Drug- or metabolic-induced nausea	2.5–5 mg
Methotrimeprazine	Nausea, agitation, confusion	50–100 mg
Midazolam	Restlessness, myoclonic jerking	10–30 mg
Hyoscine	Terminal bronchial secretions, colic	1.2–2.4 mg

however, increasing the concentration and number of drugs mixed increases the likelihood of crystallization or degradation and so no more than three or four should be mixed. Protecting the syringe contents from light helps to reduce problems with drug degradation.

During infusion the injection site should be checked regularly for signs of inflammation or infection. The syringe contents should be checked to ensure that crystallization has not occurred and that there is no leakage from the administration set or around the site of insertion. It is also essential to check that the correct volume is being delivered and that the battery has not become exhausted. For the type of pump described here (Graseby MS16 and MS26) one battery should deliver about 50 syringes, and therefore last about seven weeks. To deliver 10 ml in 24 hours, the MS16 is set to 2 mm per hour and the MS26 to 48 mm per day.

Irritation at the injection site may be due to drugs such as cyclizine and methotrimeprazine. Diazepam, prochlorperazine, and chlorpromazine are too irritant and therefore should not be given by this route. If the problem continues, it may be possible to change to less irritant drugs such as haloperidol, or to administer the original drugs by the rectal route.

Crystallization of the syringe contents may be a problem with cyclizine or haloperidol, especially when high concentrations of diamorphine are

Table 8.3 Co-analgesic drugs and their indications

Drug	Indications	Common side-effects
NSAID	Tissue destruction, inflammation, pruritus, sweating, bone erosion	GI and renal problems
Steroids	Nerve compression, raised intracranial pressure, anorexia, weight loss, pelvic invasion, cord compression, bone pain, liver distension	Increased weight, fluid retention, insomnia
Muscle relaxants	Muscle spasm	Sedation, especially with diazepam
Antidepressants	Dysaesthesia, burning, night sedation, depression	Sedation, dry mouth, urinary retention
Anticonvulsants	Lancinating, shooting pains	GI upset, blood dyscrasias
Sedatives	Agitation, restlessness	Somnolence, hypotension
Bone metabolic drugs	Bone pain	Nausea

used. If this occurs the syringe and the giving set should be changed and the volume of infusion increased to 20 ml over 24 hours. Keeping the syringe away from sunlight or heat will also reduce this problem.

Diamorphine is the analgesic of choice for subcutaneous infusion because its high solubility means that large doses can be given in small volumes. If converting from oral medication, use one third of the 24 hour oral dose of morphine or half the 24 hour oral dose of diamorphine. If this does not control the pain adequately, increase the dose in increments of 25–50 per cent. If a booster dose is required to cover breakthrough pain, then a bolus equivalent to one sixth of the daily dose can be given.

Syringe drivers are a valuable means of providing symptomatic relief. However, they are sometimes used when they are not necessary, as most patients can be managed on oral medication. The true indications for subcutaneous infusion are: nausea and vomiting; inability to swallow; unconsciousness; and poor absorption of oral medication.

Other drugs used to manage pain

Several other classes of drug may be helpful (Table 8.3), and different approaches have to be tried if pain is uncontrolled (Fig. 8.4).

NSAIDs

Their inhibitory effect on the production of the chemical mediators of inflammation makes these drugs useful as mild analgesics both alone and combined with opioid therapy to produce more effective analgesia. This may be especially helpful where tissue destruction is a factor, for example when pain is caused by metastatic deposits in bone. All NSAIDs may cause side-effects such as gastrointestinal bleeding or intolerance, even when enteric-coated preparations are used or when they are given rectally. Nevertheless, some patients tolerate diclofenac or piroxicam better as suppositories than when given orally. For patients who may already be on many different drugs there are obvious advantages in a preparation which can be given 12 hourly (such as flubiprofen 100 mg) or once daily (such as piroxicam 20 mg). NSAIDs may also be useful in the management of localized cutaneous inflammation as well as pruritus, which can be a troublesome symptom in malignant disease. They may also reduce the distressing night sweats which can occur in these patients.

Steroids

Steroid therapy can reduce pain resulting from the pressure of a tumour on surrounding tissues. Such pains arise from compression of peripheral

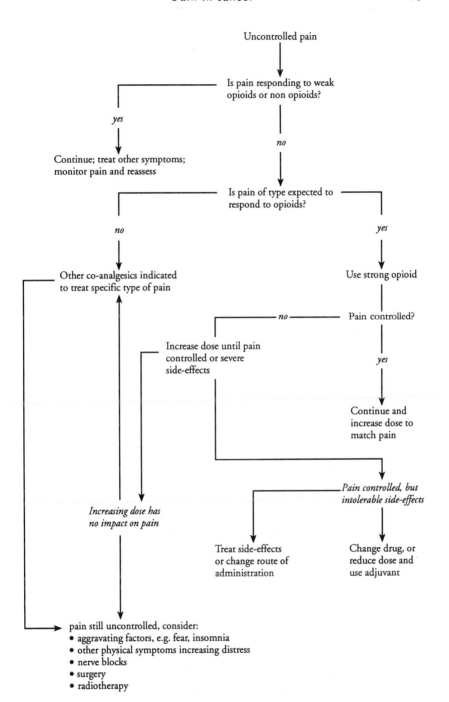

Fig. 8.4 Management of uncontrolled pain.

nerves, spinal cord compression or raised intracranial pressure, and infiltration of organs such as the liver with resulting distension of the capsule.

Dexamethasone is effective and this should be started in a high dose, initially of 12–24 mg per day. This can be given as a single dose or in three divided doses, although the last dose should be given no later than late afternoon as occasionally insomnia may be aggravated by evening doses of steroids. An effect should be evident within about two days. The dose can be reduced gradually after about a week to the lowest dose that will continue to control symptoms.

Although dexamethasone is less likely to produce unpleasant side-effects than other steroids, slight oedema may occur. Psychotic changes are rare and are reversed on stopping the drug. Improved appetite with some weight gain and a feeling of well being are beneficial side-effects of steroids for cachectic patients.

Tricyclic antidepressants

Many patients with malignant disease suffer from depression which exceeds the expected sadness resulting from their condition. Antidepressant drugs may reduce these symptoms. A drug such as lofepramine 140–210 mg per day will have less side-effects than some of the older drugs. If night-time sedation is needed, dothiepin 25–75 mg or the tetracyclic mianserin 30–90 mg at night are useful.

However, antidepressant drugs can also play an important role as analgesics. This property is only marked in a few of the tricyclic antidepressant drugs. They are used in the management of pain which has a neurogenic component, usually as a result of damage to nervous tissue, either peripherally or centrally. These pains are felt as unpleasant and abnormal sensations, such as burning or painful hypersensitivity. They include deafferentation pains resulting from functional denervation of a part of the body, some pains maintained by apparent excessive activity of the sympathetic nervous system (sympathetically maintained pain), and neuralgias resulting from toxic or destructive factors.

Neurogenic pains are usually unresponsive to clinical doses of opioid analgesics, but they may only form one component of a pain of mixed aetiology. Tricyclic drugs are therefore often administered with opioid drugs to produce better pain control than the latter can alone.

The tricyclic drug of choice for managing pain associated with unpleasant abnormal sensory changes is amitriptyline. It can cause more unpleasant side-effects than the alternatives, but it is undoubtedly the most effective. Patients should be warned of the dry mouth which almost invariably occurs. Its sedative effects may be an advantage at night, and for that reason the drug should be given as a single night-time dose. Daytime sedation may be troublesome in the ambulant patient but this frequently diminishes after the first few days and can be minimized by starting at a low dose and increasing this gradually every two or three days to the most effective dose. The anticholinergic effects of amitriptyline may cause urinary retention in patients who have a degree of prostatic enlargement, and may mean that a less anticholinergic drug has to be used instead.

Usually, amitriptyline is started at a dose of 10–25 mg at night and increased in increments of 25 mg. An analgesic effect is usually evident before any antidepressant effect, and often at lower doses. It is not usually necessary to exceed a dose of 75 mg although a few patients may need up to 150 mg. Other tricyclic antidepressants which are effective in relieving neurogenic pain are nortriptyline (which is less sedating than amitriptyline), clomipramine, desipramine, and—perhaps to a lesser extent—dothiepin and doxepin.

Anticonvulsants

Damage to nervous tissue may also generate sharp shooting or lancinating pains. This type of pain is also usually unresponsive to opioids but may respond to the anticonvulsant drugs. The most frequently used drug in this group is carbamazepine, which can be started at a dose of 100 mg at night and gradually increased until a satisfactory response is achieved. The maximum dose is 400 mg three times a day. Some patients are intolerant of carbamazepine and are unable to increase to an effective dose because of drowsiness, dizziness and disorientation, or gastrointestinal intolerance. It is then worth trying alternative preparations such as sodium valproate. Indeed, many specialists would start with valproate before trying carbamazepine. Again the starting dose might be as low as 100 mg daily, increased to a maximum of 600 mg three times a day if necessary. Sodium valproate can occasionally cause blood dyscrasias or disturbance of liver function and it is advisable occasionally to monitor these. Rarely it causes alopecia, but this is reversible on stopping the drug. Either of these drugs may be used in combination with tricyclics to manage neurogenic pain.

Clonazepam may be useful for this type of pain, and should be given as a single night-time dose starting at 500 μg and increasing to a maximum of 4 mg. However, many elderly and debilitated patients will find clonazepam is too sedative and will therefore be unable to tolerate it.

Other approaches to pain relief

Surgery

There may be no prospect of a cure by surgery, but it may still have a valuable palliative role in certain conditions. Relief of bowel obstruction by a bypass or ostomy procedure may be important where some weeks or months of life are expected even though the underlying condition cannot be arrested by surgery. When pain arises from metastases in bone, surgical fixation of actual or potential fractures may be necessary to relieve pain. Surgery should be performed before radiotherapy as it may be more difficult afterwards. Surgical decompression of the spinal cord may be necessary to relieve pain and preserve some function when metastases in the spine are compressing nervous tissue.

Radiotherapy

This may help relieve pain caused by bone metastases, nerve tissue compression, or where there is extensive soft tissue infiltration. A short course or single dose of palliative radiotherapy can produce dramatic relief of symptoms in suitable cases. The analgesic effects can appear quite rapidly, before there is any obvious reduction in tumour mass. There may be an important effect on function of cells such as osteoclasts which are locally destroying bone tissue. The advice of a radiotherapist should be sought early in the management of this type of pain.

Nerve blocking and destructive procedures

In the early days of palliative care, neurodestructive procedures played a major part in pain control. Such techniques have undergone a dramatic decline over recent years as other methods of pain relief have become more sophisticated. Much pain results from damage to nervous tissue, so the further destruction of nerves is not always the best way to deal with the problem. Destruction of nerves either by neurolytic injections or by surgical division results in loss of normal sensation and possibly loss of normal motor function and sphincter control, and may produce further unpleasant and painful sensations associated with deafferentation.

Nerve destruction is usually undertaken only when there is no other satisfactory means of controlling pain. It should be performed for a highly selective aim with minimal detrimental side-effects, and generally only when the patient's life expectancy is limited.

Peripheral nerve blocks These should ideally avoid any significant motor blockade and only be used where alternative means of analgesia are inadequate, for example where a clearly localized metastatic lesion in a rib is producing severe pain on movement. If a trial intercostal block with local anaesthetic relieves the pain, it may be justified to proceed with a nerve block using phenol to produce a long-lasting effect. Such a procedure is, however, unlikely to provide permanent relief and the patient may develop a painful neuritic pain to replace the original one.

Segmental nerves can be blocked in the paravertebral space to relieve pain arising in the body wall tissues of the chest and abdomen, and may occasionally be helpful with pain that is predominantly nociceptive in origin (arising as a result of continuing damage in the tissues) rather than neuropathic pain arising from damage to nerve tissue.

Again, temporary block with local anaesthetic should be performed to assess the effect of the nerve blockade. If this produces good relief, a more permanent effect can be achieved by repeating the block with aqueous phenol. The procedure is not without risk because the phenol may spread intradurally and cause widespread damage to the nervous system. There is also the possibility of producing a painful neuritis in the distribution of the blocked nerve and, in the longer term, deafferentation pain. However, in appropriate cases nerve blockade can greatly improve symptom control.

Where nociceptive pain is clearly limited to a single nerve root and relief of pain can be demonstrated with a local anaesthetic block, a lesion may be made in the dorsal root ganglion of that nerve to relieve pain. Under radiological control an electrode needle is placed close to the ganglion where it lies in the intervertebral foramen, and a radiofrequency alternating current produces a thermal lesion in the sensory fibres of the nerve. This requires specialized equipment, and the patient has to be able to tolerate an uncomfortable procedure.

Occasionally the sacral nerves are blocked to relieve intractable perineal pain. A needle is inserted into the sacral foramen. The relief of pain can be dramatic but again the procedure should only be undertaken when no suitable alternatives are possible and when life expectancy is very limited. Impairing sphincter control is a major hazard of blocking sacral nerves.

Subarachnoid and epidural blockade Neurolytic substances (usually phenol or alcohol) were once often injected into the subarachnoid space to relieve pain in cancer. In the early days of pain specialists, this was one of the few means available for providing good relief of intractable pain, and the results were often dramatic in patients for whom no other relief seemed possible. Indications for this procedure are now much less frequent, since alternative analgesic techniques have become available, and because the side-effects of neurolytic blockade, such as motor paralysis and incontinence, are potentially so detrimental to the patient's well-being. Nevertheless, there are occasions when pain control is extremely difficult, life expectancy is poor and sphincter control may already be lost. In these situations subarachnoid block can produce very effective relief for a patient whose quality of life is already very poor.

Subarachnoid block can be done more accurately, and therefore more safely, with the help of an image intensifier. However, there are a few situations when it is justified to perform it as a bedside technique to bring dramatic pain relief to a debilitated patient towards the end of life.

For subarachnoid block, phenol is usually administered in glycerol which makes it heavier than CSF. The injection is performed with the patient lying on the side to be blocked, as the phenol will tend to settle on the dependent nerve roots. If alcohol is used, the patient is positioned with the painful side uppermost, as the alcohol tends to rise in the CSF. Hyperbaric phenol has the advantage of a slightly more predictable spread within the subarachnoid space and is less likely to produce painful neuritis after the injection.

The needle is inserted under local anaesthesia into the subarachnoid space where the neurolytic solution is injected. In the lumbar region there is a risk of the solution spreading to the sacral nerve roots, causing loss of sphincter control. This risk is minimized by keeping the volume of solution very small and repeating the injection a few days later if pain is not adequately relieved.

Injections are sometimes given into the epidural space, but this approach remains less popular as the distribution of the block may be more difficult to control than with the subarachnoid route.

If pain is poorly controlled by parenteral drugs, or a patient cannot tolerate the doses of drugs needed for pain control, injections or infusions of local anaesthetics or opioids (or both) are sometimes given into the epidural space. A catheter is inserted percutaneously into the epidural space and either used for intermittent injection or, more commonly, connected to an infusion device. If the infusion is to be continued for more than a few days the catheter can be tunnelled subcutaneously so that it exits from the skin away from the site of entry to the spine, so reducing the risk of introducing infection into the epidural space. Infusion can be either by a small battery operated syringe driver (as used for subcutaneous infusions), or from a reservoir containing sufficient drug for many days.

Alternatively when it is anticipated that the epidural drugs will be used for some time, a reservoir with subcutaneous injection port can be implanted. Epidural diamorphine or morphine will provide analgesia at far smaller doses than would be required parenterally and so with fewer systemic side-effects such as sedation. The combined use of low dose bupivacaine and diamorphine infused into the epidural space may be a useful means of providing relief from pain on movement associated with skeletal metastases. The insertion and maintenance of such devices requires experienced medical and nursing staff if they are to be safe and effective.

Autonomic blockade   The coeliac plexus lies anterior to the bodies of the first lumbar and the twelfth thoracic vertebrae and through it pass efferent and afferent sympathetic fibres from the upper abdominal viscera. Destruction of tracts passing through the coeliac plexus may relieve pain arising from the pancreas, liver, kidneys, and stomach. This is one of the few destructive procedures which can be indicated soon after a malignant disease of these organs has been diagnosed and when pain control starts to become a problem. It will often relieve virtually all the pain from such conditions. Even if it does not relieve it completely, it often makes it easier to control with analgesic drugs.

Coeliac plexus block is a percutaneous injection procedure but it must be performed under radiological control using an image intensifier. The injection is painful, so it is necessary either to use adequate local anaesthesia plus some sedation, or to perform the procedure under a light general anaesthetic, which may be more acceptable to the patient.

Needles are inserted bilaterally below the twelfth rib to lie anterior to the upper part of the body of the first lumbar vertebra. Absolute alcohol is diluted with local anaesthetic and a total volume of 30–40 ml is injected, divided between the two sides.

Coeliac plexus block causes a sympathetic block which may result in postural hypotension. This is usually self-limiting and it should be managed in the early stages with adequate fluid intake and if necessary with elastic compression stockings. The effects of coeliac plexus block often wane after a few months and it may be necessary to repeat the procedure.

Lumbar sympathetic block   Blocking the lumbar sympathetic chain may relieve rest pain and improve skin perfusion in patients with peripheral vascular disease. However, the sympathetic system also has a role in maintaining painful states following nerve damage (autonomic dystrophies) and may be involved in the perception of some pain arising in the lower abdominal and pelvic viscera. Lumbar sympathetic block may therefore be helpful when pain arises in these areas as a result of malignant disease. It will not help when pain arises from skeletal tissue or invasion of pelvic nerves.

The lumbar sympathetic ganglia lie retroperitoneally along the anterolateral borders of the lumbar vertebrae. Using an image intensifier, a needle can be placed in the fascial compartment in which these ganglia lie, and a neurolytic solution, usually phenol, injected. The procedure can easily be performed under local anaesthesia, perhaps using light sedation. The most likely complication is the development of postural hypotension, but this is rarely a problem. Occasionally there is some spread of neurolytic solution onto the lower lumbar sensory nerves which can cause burning pain in the groin and upper thigh. This is usually minimal and self-limiting if the correct procedure is followed.

Cordotomy   When pain signals are processed in the spinal cord, much of the information travels up to the higher centres of the nervous system by crossing to the contralateral side of the spinal cord and through the anterolateral spinothalamic tract. It is possible to prevent the sensation of pain arising in one side of the body by interrupting this tract. The tract can be surgically cut or, as is now more common, interrupted by inserting an electrode into the tract under radiological control and producing a thermal lesion. This relieves pain in all areas below the level of the lesion on the opposite side of the body.

Producing such a lesion in the CNS will not permanently abolish pain as the nervous system adapts to 'accommodate' the block and the pain eventually returns, often in a more unpleasant and intractable form (see Chapter 2). However, the technique is often very effective in relieving severe unilateral pain in patients whose life expectancy is not likely to outlast the period of effective blockade (up to about a year). Specialized equipment and skills are necessary but appropriate cases can usually be referred to a centre where the procedure is practised with sufficient frequency and the skills and facilities are available.

The final days

Towards the end of life, the administration of medication can present some new problems. Impairment of consciousness and difficulties in swallowing or absorption may make the use of oral medication impossible. When treatment is entirely palliative, many drugs can be discontinued and yet it is essential to continue with others. It will usually be necessary to continue to give analgesics, as sudden withdrawal may produce unpleasant symptoms. In any case a semiconscious patient will still need to be kept pain free, especially when communication is becoming difficult. Opioid analgesics can be continued by subcutaneous infusion, and if necessary, antiemetics and sedatives can be included. Other drugs affecting the cardiovascular, respiratory, and gastrointestinal systems can generally be stopped at this stage. The accumulation of respiratory secretions in the pharynx can often be distressing, particularly to relatives, and this can be controlled with a small dose of subcutaneous hyoscine.

The care of dying patients involves far more than the relief of pain. Many other symptoms may require attention, as well as the psychological, social, and spiritual care of the dying. These aspects are beyond the scope of this book and the interested reader is referred to the list of further reading.

Further reading

Doyle, D., Hanks, G. W. C., and Macdonald, N. (1993). *Oxford textbook of palliative medicine*. Oxford University Press, Oxford.

Oliver, D. J. (1988). Syringe drivers in palliative care: a review. *Palliative Medicine*, 2, 21-6.

Regnard, C. F. B. and Tempest, S. (1992). *A guide to symptom relief in advanced cancer.* Haigh and Hochland, Manchester.

Saunders, C. H. (ed.) (1978). *The management of terminal disease.* Edward Arnold, London.

Twycross, R. G. and Lack, S. A. (1983). *Symptom control in advanced cancer: pain relief.* Pitman, London.

9 *Pain as a long-term problem*

Chronic pain and the pain clinic
Pathology and chronic pain syndromes
The management of chronic pain

Pain is useful. It tells us that we have injured ourselves. We can ignore pain that is not severe enough to affect our enjoyment or quality of life when we are assured that it is not caused by a disease or injury. If it is caused by a disease or injury and it goes when the cause is cured, the pain is now no longer of any significance. All other pains are significant. They generate suffering, they cause anxiety and then depression. They interfere with the ability to live a normal life. They cause invalidity. These pains are part of chronic disease. In the absence of a causative disease, the pain becomes a disease.

Conventionally we consider a disease to be the result of a disorder of bodily function, which causes symptoms and signs. Disease is that which causes ill health and ill health is experienced when changes in the mind or body make it no longer possible to enjoy life as a healthy person would. Where pain is experienced as a result of a lesion of the body or mind that we can identify we accept that pain as a symptom of disease and, in part, value it as an aid to diagnosis and an indicator as to how the disease might be cured. When pain is being felt in the absence of any diagnosable lesion of the body or mind, it must still be the result of a disorder of function.

If pain is experienced when there is no tissue damage then the disorder must lie in the system of pain perception, a system that should be differentiating between the painful and the not painful. In Chapter 3 we described the psychological processes that are associated with pain and the learning processes that generate pain behaviour. If disordered behaviour that generates ill health fulfils our definition of disease, then at some point malingering becomes self-fulfilling. It becomes a disease.

Chronic pain and the pain clinic

Between seven and ten per cent of the population of the UK suffers from chronic pain. Nearly half of all disabled people have severe unrelieved pain, even though there is a complex system for curing disease available in the UK and everywhere else in the economically advanced world. This means that however advanced a medical system, its impact on the global pain problem is inadequate.

It has become clear that much chronic pain can be lessened if the symptom is given sufficient skilled and specialist attention. In addition, if the problems of chronic pain are understood and correctly managed, the resulting invalidity can be greatly reduced.

It has become increasingly clear that the management of pain which is not relieved by simple means requires special knowledge and skill. Thus, as in all branches of science, specialization has developed; the best results in managing pain will come to those who take a special interest in its physiology, pathology, and pharmacology, and its psychological consequences. Specialization in medicine has always been criticized. The specialist has, sometimes justifiably, been described as the doctor who knows more and more about less and less. However, the specialist in pain management who fulfilled this gloomy definition would be a dangerous person indeed. The dangers of symptomatic treatment are abundantly clear. Pain is a symptom of damage and neglecting its warnings can lead to progressive injury, or even death.

Specialists in pain management will always be aware that back pain can be, though rarely is, a symptom of infectious, neoplastic, or other damaging disease. Their history taking and physical examination must always be scrupulous. If there are symptoms or signs which raise any suspicions of underlying disease a specialist must always be ready to refer the patient for assessment by people with other skills.

Where pain presents a problem and has become apparently intractable, specialist treatment stands the best chance of understanding its cause, lessening its impact, and minimizing the disability that it might cause. This is the function of a pain clinic.

The nature of chronic pain

It is important to understand the effect that persistent pain will have upon the sufferer. When deformity and stiffness in a limb are caused by arthritis, or sight or hearing is damaged by the loss of function of an eye or an ear, the relationship between the failed function and the cause is clear. The symptom of pain causes disability without an associated cause being evident. The sufferer from phantom limb pain has no limb there to hurt, the patient with post-herpetic neuralgia no longer has shingles, and sufferers from post-stroke central pain have had their strokes. There is no obvious damage to tissue or disease which might be causing these pains. People who suffer from only occasional pains, which then go, find it almost impossible to imagine perpetual pain.

To suffer from such pain generates behavioural change. It is not the pain itself that results in the patient being an invalid, it is the sufferer's reaction to the pain. Society reinforces the situation through the reaction of people around the patient to the outward indicators of pain. The facial expressions, other body movements that indicate pain and discomfort, and verbal complaints of pain generate a need to help and support the sufferer and this reinforces the invalid role.

One human has no idea of what another feels. We therefore believe that others are feeling what we believe they should be feeling. A patient who has had a small operation should not have as much pain as a patient who has had a large operation. When someone has had too much to drink they should have a headache. A broken leg hurts a lot. If someone has no disease or injury they should have no pain.

In truth, we can never know whether someone else is in pain or not. We have no reason or right to believe that someone who says that they are in pain is not in pain. The acknowledgement of the pain is frequently one of the most valuable things that a pain clinician or anyone else involved with a sufferer from chronic pain can offer.

The role of clinics

Patients with pain that persists in spite of all therapy to cure any disease that may be causing it, and patients who have pain in the absence of diagnosed disease are likely to become unnecessarily disabled. Referral for specialist help from a pain clinic will reduce this disability and may reduce or relieve their pain.

The skills needed to deal with chronic pain come from several disciplines. Among the problems that develop in patients with chronic sickness are an over-dependence on doctors, a belief that somewhere is a medical solution if only it can be found, and a tendency to confer onto others the control of their lives. Much of these patients' invalidity is of no value to them. They need to regain a dependence on themselves to control their own lives and symptoms. They must be taught to cope with the unrelievable pain and to function in society. Psychologists, physiotherapists, occupational therapists, and nurses with a specialist interest in pain management should undertake this part of pain management. They are trained in rehabilitation and the psychological management of disability, and they help patients to realize that the best solution to their problems is not medical but lies in an understanding of the nature of their pain and in learning how to alter their behaviour so as to lessen the disability which results. The staff of a pain clinic must therefore be multidisciplinary and each discipline should have its own place in the patient's management.

Sources of referral

Symptomatic treatment of pain in the first instance is wrong. A sick person should first be put through a systematic process of investigation. If this has been competently and completely done and the sufferer continues to complain of pain then a referral to a pain clinic is indicated. The usual pattern is that 45 per cent of referrals are from general practitioners and 55 per cent from other specialists. Some clinics will only accept referrals from specialists, but we feel this is a mistake and results in needless delay. Any competent clinician can identify the patients who meet the criteria for referral, and any pain specialist should be able to assess whether patients have been referred appropriately or whether they need a different type of help.

Self-referral could be disastrous, as 85 per cent of all patients who seek medical help do so because of pain. In most, the cause of the pain is self-limiting, and in most of the rest the cause can be treated and the pain relieved.

Aims and results of a pain clinic

Are specialist services for pain justified? The only outcome that patients would regard as satisfactory would be relief from their pain, and this should be the first object of a pain clinic. All pain clinic patients have difficult problems but, in spite of this, most clinics will relieve pain in between 30 and 40 per cent of their patients. In a further 20 per cent pain is reduced, and almost all feel that they have benefited from coming to a pain clinic because of the attention to and acknowledgement of their pain.

Rehabilitative measures are much more successful. Most pain management groups produce major reductions in invalid behaviour, drug consumption, and demand for medical and social services in around 85 per cent of patients they see.

Pathology and chronic pain syndromes

Diseases that are painful and incurable will of course cause chronic pain. Cancer is the most feared of these, but inflammatory or degenerative arthritis can cause pain as severe as cancer that lasts for very much longer. CNS diseases that interfere with the processing of sensory function can cause chronic pain syndromes, and are a more common cause of unrelieved pain than is usually acknowledged. Half of people with multiple sclerosis suffer from chronic pain, 2 per cent of stroke patients develop central post-stroke pain, and spinal cord injury usually results in chronic pain.

Peripheral nerve damage may cause pain, and the longer the damage persists, the more likely it is to cause pain. For example, diabetic and other chronic neuropathies are painless initially, but become painful after a time. Post-herpetic neuralgia is the result of both peripheral and central damage. In younger patients, the nervous system has enough reserve and plasticity to replace the sensory functions that are lost when the varicella virus emerges from the dorsal horn neurons in which it has been living and destroys both the neurone and its axon. Plasticity decreases with age, and the incidence of post-herpetic neuralgia increases, rising to 60 per cent of cases of herpes zoster in people over 70.

The cause of sympathetic dystrophy is still debated. It is possible that the initial disturbance is a behavioural one. It may be that the condition starts because the affected part is over-protected from use and sensory input following injury. It cannot be induced in experimental animals without producing much grosser interferences with nerve function than are found in humans with the condition. The initial change, of hypersensitivity to light touch, is followed by marked physical changes, with an alteration in blood flow, bone resorption, changes in nail and hair growth, and eventually atrophy. The manifestations of sympathetic dystrophy are so disparate that there is still a debate between those who are unconvinced that it exists, and those who believe it to be present in any pain which is relieved by sympathetic blockade.

The management of chronic pain

The management of chronic pain is complex and needs specialist intervention. All those caring for people who are ill should recognize and acknowledge the existence of pain and the need to provide appropriate help. Pain needs to be treated with drugs that provide a continuous level of relief, rather than brief pain-free windows and long painful interludes. Sufferers who are withdrawing from a working, social, and sexual life, and making inappropriate use of wheelchairs, crutches, and medication should be encouraged to reject any aids that are not absolutely essential. The illness behaviour that results from unrelieved pain is learned. It is vital that medical and nursing staff do not initiate or reinforce this maladaptive learning.

10 *Musculoskeletal pain*

The largest group of patients presenting with symptoms of pain suffer from some form of musculoskeletal pain. Some causes of musculoskeletal pain and disability are related to clearly defined diseases, for example inflammatory disease such as rheumatoid arthritis, or well recognized metabolic or degenerative conditions such as osteoarthritis or osteoporosis. Everyone at some time in their lives suffers from various aches and pains for which no cause can be diagnosed. Most of these resolve spontaneously, but in some people they progress to a chronic state resulting in long-term suffering and disability. Failure to identify a causative lesion frequently leads to the pain and suffering being dismissed by the medical profession as a 'supratentorial' problem. This is a medical euphemism for imagined pain. It is, however, rare to meet a doctor who has experienced imaginary pain and can describe the experience! The poor record of help from established medicine for many sufferers from these conditions has led them to try some of the many alternative treatments in this area.

Osteoarthritis

Osteoarthritis, or osteoarthrosis, is one of the commonest afflictions of humans. It affects most elderly people to some degree, and it is prevalent in all parts of the world. There is good archaeological evidence of the widespread incidence of degenerative joint disease in all previous societies. However, although joint degeneration is almost universal, pain and disability are not. It is difficult to understand the poor correlation between pain and radiological or pathological evidence of joint degeneration. Often joints that appear badly damaged on X-ray examination cause very few symptoms, and joints with little damage may be very painful. Younger age groups are not always spared the pain of degenerative joint disease.

Osteoarthritis is characterized by a process of degradation of the articular cartilage with increased density of the subchondral bone. Osteophytes and bone cysts frequently develop. There may be a low-grade synovitis of the affected joints and the sufferer frequently experiences a deep aching pain, which may be poorly localized, as well as stiffness and pain on movement. This is usually worse on waking and tends to ease with activity. Night pain is common. The hands, knees, hips, shoulders, and spine are most frequently affected. When osteoarthritis of the spine affects the discs and facet joints (apophyseal joints) it is termed spondylosis. This may be responsible for much back and neck pain, but again the radiological evidence of disease is often poorly correlated with symptoms. When nerve roots are affected by the development of osteophytes or the narrowing of intervertebral foramina by arthritic facet joints, there will be symptoms of nerve root compression as well.

Joint replacement surgery has been extremely successful in relieving pain and reducing disability. However, when surgical replacement of joints is not possible, or the condition is not regarded as being severe enough to justify major surgery, symptomatic management is usually the only option. The pain and stiffness of an arthritic joint can often be effectively relieved by intra-articular injections of corticosteroids. The shoulder, knee and apophyseal joints of the spine are particularly amenable to this treatment. However, the benefits are limited and there is concern that frequent intra-articular injections may cause long-term damage to joints.

Blocking the nerve supply to a painful joint with local anaesthetic will often provide surprisingly prolonged relief, and this may be applied to the spinal joints, the hip and shoulder joints in particular. It was originally thought that the method brought relief by reducing periarticular muscle spasm, but it is difficult to account fully for the prolonged pain relief in this way. It is probable that the pain from an arthritic joint depends on an afferent nerve supply which is blocked by local anaesthetic. Local anaesthetic blocks may reduce the input of nociception to the CNS, so reducing the enhanced level of neuronal activity believed to exist in chronic pain. Specific nerve block for these joints is technically difficult and is outside the scope of this book.

The pain and stiffness of degenerate joints is often relieved by acupuncture. Hips and knees seem to be particularly amenable, providing there is no major disorganization of the joint. With a basic knowledge of acupuncture techniques it is possible to help relieve this type of pain.

Most people suffering from degenerative joint disease rely on the use of analgesic drugs and general supportive measures. Non-steroidal anti-inflammatory drugs (NSAIDs) are often the first-line treatment. A long-acting NSAID taken orally or by suppository before retiring to bed will often help relieve night pain and morning stiffness. Many patients who benefit may be maintained on these drugs for long periods. However, many patients obtain only short-term or no relief from NSAIDs, and these drugs are associated with a relatively high incidence of side-effects. Gastrointestinal irritation frequently makes them intolerable, and they are contraindicated in patients with peptic ulceration, asthma, renal impairment or allergy to any similar drugs.

Simple analgesics may provide effective relief. Paracetamol is popular, either alone or in combination with one of the weak opioids such as codeine. Again, many patients cease to gain relief after a time, but continue to consume large quantities as nothing else seems to be available. Providing that the dose limits for paracetamol are adhered to, the long-term use of such drugs seems to be relatively harmless. However, an attempt should be made to establish that they do help pain or mobility before continuing to prescribe them. Nefopam is an alternative drug which can be tried in those patients who appear to benefit from analgesic therapy, but who are unable to tolerate paracetamol or weak opioids.

Most patients who suffer from degenerative joint disease either do not benefit greatly from opioids, or find the side-effects intolerable. Nevertheless, when other drugs and therapies have failed to relieve pain and improve mobility, and if the quality of life is badly affected, a controlled regular dose of long-acting opioid can occasionally be helpful. This may be especially effective for night pain in the elderly, allowing the sufferer a good night's sleep. However side-effects may severely restrict the use of opioids in these patients and they should only be used if they clearly benefit symptoms.

The stiffness and immobility that accompany degenerate joint disease contribute to further pain and distress. Physiotherapists can give valuable help in managing the pain, by mobilizing stiff joints and developing an exercise programme suited to the patient, which they can then continue at home.

Inflammatory arthritis

The inflammatory arthritic conditions are a group of usually well defined diseases. They have their own specific treatments, which are beyond the scope of this book. Care is often a team effort involving the primary care team, rheumatologist, orthopaedic surgeon, rehabilitation specialists, occupational therapists, and physiotherapists. Physical means of relieving disability may help to relieve the pain, but many patients still have pain as a major symptom. NSAIDs, including salicylates, are frequently used. These can be effective but their use may be restricted by gastrointestinal side-effects, liver or renal damage, or coexisting asthma. Steroids are used in severe cases, either systemically or intra-articularly, but these may also have long-term deleterious effects. Disease-modifying drugs such as gold, penicillamine, antimalarials, and immunosuppressives, and surgery to stabilize disorganized joints may help to reduce pain. Rarely, sympathetic nerve blocks help.

However, most patients are managed with simple analgesics such as paracetamol, alone or in combination with weak opioid drugs like di-hydrocodeine. Pain which responds to analgesic drugs may sometimes be severe enough to justify the use of regular oral potent opioid analgesics, although given the long-term nature of the condition, many doctors are reluctant to embark on this course. Where other measures have failed to control pain adequately, and where a clear improvement in pain control can be demonstrated without unacceptable side-effects, the use of oral morphine may be considered.

Myofascial pain and fibromyalgia

There is a group of painful conditions of muscle and connective tissue which have been variously recognized (or not recognized) by the medical profession over the past century, and which have been given a great number of different names. The conditions are difficult to define, difficult to differentiate, and attempts to demonstrate an underlying pathophysiology have been unproductive. Although many would claim that these conditions are responsible for much chronic pain and disability, the failure to demonstrate consistent pathological changes in the painful tissues has led many doctors to deny their physical reality.

Nevertheless, patients suffering from these conditions constitute a large proportion of those referred to pain management services and it seems that they are responsible for much pain and disability in the population. Names such as muscular rheumatism, myositis, myofascitis, fibrositis, and fibromyalgia have been used, but these suggest a false understanding of the causes. Fibromyalgia and myofascial syndrome are now the most commonly used terms and are recognized as such by the Committee on Taxonomy of the International Association for the Study of Pain.

Fibromyalgia

Fibromyalgia is a chronic condition characterized by diffuse muscle stiffness and tenderness, usually in at least twelve recognized sites. There may be articular pain with a subjective impression of swelling of the extremities. There is sometimes a sensation of coldness in the limbs with occasional reticular skin discolouration. There is a chronic pattern of non-restorative sleep, with a decrease of non-rapid eye movement (REM) sleep and changes in the EEG which are almost diagnostic. Patients generally complain of fatigue, stiffness, variable paraesthesiae and subjective muscle tension, but all radiological and laboratory studies are usually within normal limits.

The symptoms may develop following an episode of trauma (such as the chronic pain following a 'whiplash injury') or may have a more gradual onset. Repetitive strain resulting from poor working postures seems to be a factor in the development of the condition in some individuals, and emotional stress also seems to be involved. Episodes of acute or repetitive mechanical overload of the affected muscles may be a factor in the development of both fibromyalgia and myofascial pain syndromes.

The intensity of symptoms varies but often there is no permanent relief and the condition may be lifelong. Chronic headache, irritable bowel syndrome, and Raynaud's disease are frequently associated with fibromyalgia. The median age of onset of symptoms seems to be 29–37 and female sufferers outnumber males. There may be as many as 6 million sufferers in the USA and up to 20 per cent of patients referred to rheumatology clinics may be affected. However, because of variable acceptance and diagnosis of fibromyalgia and related conditions, the true incidence is difficult to verify.

Myofascial pain syndrome

The myofascial pain syndrome is differentiated from primary fibromyalgia by the existence of tender areas of muscle (or other soft tissue). Palpation of these 'trigger-points' reproduces the pain, although it is often referred to a distant area. The pattern of pain referred from trigger points is predictable and reproducible although it does not follow strict dermatomal patterns. The patient is often not aware of the existence of trigger points, only experiencing the referred pain, but it is usually easy to predict where the trigger points will be found from the patient's description of pain distribution. The trigger points may be well defined, but sometimes seem to be a band of muscle. There is a strong correlation between well defined trigger points and many traditional acupuncture points.

Myofascial pain shares with fibromyalgia the features of disturbance of normal sleep patterns and a lack of convincingly demonstrable pathology in the affected tissues. The two conditions may be variations of the same syndrome and it is not always possible to separate them completely.

Possible mechanisms

Many attempts have been made to identify a histological abnormality in the region of the trigger points. Biopsies will sometimes show a degree of oedema in the muscle fibres and an increase in mast cells has been reported. Generalized degenerative changes, a generally 'moth-eaten' appearance of the muscle filaments, and abnormal mitochondria can be seen microscopically. However, none of these findings are consistent or diagnostic. There seems to be some abnormal function of the muscle fibres but electromyographic studies have failed to demonstrate abnormal muscle tension. It has been suggested that there is an abnormality in local blood supply resulting in tissue hypoxia. Several neurotransmitters have been implicated in these syndromes, and 5-HT (serotonin) depletion and abnormally low levels of substance P have been proposed as underlying factors. The possibility of this being an autoimmune condition has also been examined.

Fibromyalgia may be a primary phenomenon with no obvious cause. It may, however, be secondary to other musculoskeletal conditions such as rheumatoid arthritis, ankylosing spondylitis, osteoarthritis or spinal disc degenerative conditions, and greatly increase the resulting pain and disability.

The most common sites of pain and muscle tenderness are the shoulder girdle muscles, the head, and neck and lumbar muscles. Often, several different regions are involved simultaneously. Fibromyalgia is more common in sedentary workers, although not exclusively so, and often appears to be worse in cold, damp weather.

Patients may not be aware of the muscle involvement in a myofascial pain syndrome and can present with headache, backache, sciatica, or abdominal pain. They have often been extensively investigated with negative results for disease in other systems. Examination of the area in which trigger points are commonly found will often provoke this referred pain. When the muscles are palpated with the flat surface of the examiner's finger, the patient will often jump and exclaim when the trigger point is palpated. Pain may also be referred to the usual area of symptoms at this time. Often a palpable 'nodule' or a tense band can be felt.

Treatment

Myofascial pain syndromes and fibromyalgia may cause long-term intractable symptoms, but treatment will sometimes be extremely effective, especially where there are well defined trigger points. Management generally falls into three categories: trigger point treatment, general physical methods, and medication.

Once the trigger points have been identified, they can be deactivated by direct stimulation. It has been found that the repeated injection of local anaesthetic, or local anaesthetic and steroid, or even of saline into the trigger points will give a period of relief from myofascial pain. Alternatively 'dry needling'—the insertion of a fine needle into the trigger point—will deactivate the points. As the needle enters the trigger point the patient usually experiences a sharp pain. Following treatment, the trigger point may no longer be identifiable. Unfortunately, the symptoms and the trigger points often reappear, so it is usual to give a course of treatments in order to obtain lasting relief. An alternative is the 'spray and stretch' method, in which the painful muscle is anaesthetized with a cold spray and then gently stretched.

As an adjunct to this treatment, there may be some benefit in providing other modes of physiotherapy, such as massage, heat or cold, and active and passive exercise. Usually maintaining physical fitness and exercise are emphasized although it is not easy to prove that this is effective. Transcutaneous nerve stimulation (TENS) may help to relieve symptoms in some subjects, especially in the more diffuse pain of fibromyalgia, but some patients find that this tends to aggravate their symptoms.

Analgesic drugs are usually of no help in myofascial pain and fibromyalgia, although patients may consume them in large quantities in a desperate effort to obtain relief. Occasionally the NSAIDs are helpful, but again they may be consumed more in hope than with real benefit. Tricyclic antidepressant drugs such as amitriptyline or doxepin, when taken as a single night-time dose, help to restore restful sleep and reduce morning pain and stiffness. They may also have some effect on levels of 5-HT, disturbances of which have been suggested as one of the causative factors of pain in these syndromes.

Back pain

Most people suffer from back pain at some time during their lives. In the majority, this is a self-limiting condition, often occurring after an identifiable episode of trauma or repetitive strain. A brief period of rest and analgesia followed by a gradual return to normal activity results in a resolution of the pain, although further episodes are common.

In some patients, the pain does not completely resolve, or episodes become so frequent that it becomes a chronic condition. This ranges from being a continuing source of discomfort to a condition causing severe pain and physical disability, with resulting loss of employment and normal domestic and social activities. The size of the problem seems to be increasing. It is estimated that in the UK some 52.6 million working days are lost each year because of back pain, and it is the reason for about 2.4 million medical consultations and treatments. The cost to the economy is enormous.

The cause and the most effective means of treating back pain are poorly understood. The therapies applied are legion, as are the types of therapist, whether medical, paramedical, or alternative or complementary. Each group of therapists may claim to understand the causes of back pain and therefore to be able to apply the most effective treatment. Pain often responds to some of these therapies, thus confirming the practitioner's belief in their own theory. However, the diversity of therapies suggest there is still an underlying ignorance of the nature of back pain.

Modern medicine has a need to apply a pathological label to all 'diseases', and doctors tend to suspect the authenticity of symptoms when a pathological cause cannot be found. Symptoms are attributed to abnormal behaviour or personality characteristics of the patient when a medical disease model, based on existing knowledge, fails to provide an explanation for the symptoms.

Back pain, sciatica, lumbago, and all the other synonyms and related symptoms have long been recognized, but it was with the discovery of disc prolapse and the surgery to treat it, that back pain started to acquire pathological labels. It was discovered that severe back pain and sciatica may accompany herniation of intervertebral discs. Surgery to remove the herniated portions of disc often results in resolution of the pain and other symptoms. It was therefore concluded that the 'slipped disc' must be the cause of back pain, and treatment by surgical removal or manipulation to allow the disc to 'slip back' became popular. Unfortunately many patients do not experience pain relief following technically successful surgery, and others have only short-term relief.

It is even more difficult to correlate cause and effect when modern imaging techniques fail to reveal evidence of disc prolapse or nerve root compression in patients whose symptoms and signs tend to suggest this as a cause. Evidence from these techniques has reduced unnecessary surgery, but leaves the causes of much back pain more difficult to understand.

Alternative causes of back pain include degenerative arthritis of the spinal joints. Most of the population eventually have radiological evidence of this, but not all of them will suffer from chronic back pain. Many people who do suffer from chronic back pain will have minimal or no radiological evidence of joint degeneration. Back pain may be a muscular problem and many people with chronic back pain suffer from tender muscles in the back. This often has many of the features of myofascial syndrome. However, we do not know if the muscle pain is a primary problem or secondary to underlying spinal problems and results of treatment are unpredictable and difficult to relate to definite diagnostic signs.

Non-medical therapists suggest many other causes of back pain, involving different aspects of spinal balance, movement, and posture, and they use various manipulative and physical treatments. However, the theories seem to rely on the results of such treatments for their justification rather than verifiable scientific explanations. Perhaps we should not regard chronic back pain as a disease, and should avoid all physical interventions, concentrating rather on restoration of normal function and on the behavioural and cognitive aspects of management, to lessen the resulting disability.

Acute back pain

Acute back pain is pain that arises suddenly and lasts for up to about two weeks. It may follow an episode of physical stress or may have no apparent preceding cause. There may be a longer term combination of causative factors, such as repetitive strain or postural abnormalities. Most acute injuries should be healing within about two weeks. Failure to resolve rapidly at this stage may signal the onset of subacute (up to three months) or chronic back pain. The traditional treatment is bed rest and analgesics. Much of the pain at this stage is caused by muscle spasm and the combination of a muscle relaxant with an analgesic is usually beneficial. NSAIDs are useful although when pain is severe there is some indication for combining these with an opioid drug for a short period.

Diazepam is often added as a muscle relaxant and it may be of some benefit in promoting rest in an anxious and uncomfortable patient initially. However, many patients remain on diazepam for far too long, which may lead to dependence. Muscle relaxants such as baclofen or methocarbamol may be preferable when sedative and anxiolytic effects of a benzodiazepine are not considered necessary.

Most episodes of acute back pain resolve with this approach. However, bed rest is often overused. There is no good evidence that it has any benefit for longer than two or three days. On the contrary, excessive immobilization may lead to the development of a chronic state of pain and disability. After the initial few days of rest and analgesia gradual mobilization should be encouraged, if necessary with the guidance of a physiotherapist, to promote a return to normal muscle tone and activity. Chiropractic or osteopathic manipulation may be beneficial at this stage. Immobilized muscles become stiff, shortened, and painful, and these changes may persist long after the original injury should have healed.

In some cases of acute back pain there may be symptoms and signs of nerve root compression. Where there is reason to believe that there is root compression, longer periods of rest may be justified. If there is evidence of spinal cord compression with sphincter disturbance, bilateral pain, and perineal anaesthesia, urgent decompressive surgery is indicated. Signs suggesting nerve root compression which do not resolve after a period of rest should be investigated by a CT (computerized axial tomography) scan or MRI (magnetic resonance imaging). If a disc has prolapsed and is causing nerve root compression, and if the symptoms and signs correlate well with the radiological findings, surgery may relieve the pain. However, some patients may be left with residual back pain despite the technically successful relief of nerve root compression.

If there are symptoms of nerve root compression, but the physical and radiological findings are not conclusive, or it is felt that the degree of prolapse is insufficient to warrant immediate surgical intervention, the patient may benefit from injections of local anaesthetic and slow-release steroid preparations into the epidural space. This can be easily performed by a skilled person, and can be repeated on an out-patient basis if necessary. The steroids probably relieve some of the oedema and possible inflammatory changes around nerve roots which have been compressed during the acute phase. The pain relief and muscle relaxant effects of the local anaesthetic improve mobilization and reduce the period of rest which is enforced by excessive pain. Many patients in hospital can be started on a graded exercise programme following an epidural injection and discharged. Further injections may be given over the subsequent weeks with the patient attending hospital for a few hours only on each occasion. An active programme of physiotherapy is important to enable such patients to return to normal back strength and activity.

There is no evidence that epidural injections influence the long-term outlook for back pain sufferers, but facilitation of early mobilization is valuable in preventing the problem becoming chronic. Steroid epidurals seem to be more beneficial in cases where there are clear symptoms of nerve root involvement, rather than with back pain alone, although they may provide helpful relief of pain and spasm in patients with back pain alone.

Chronic back pain

When back pain has persisted for more than three months it may be considered as a chronic condition. Once it has been established that there is no acute disc lesion producing the symptoms, and providing that specific pathologies such as primary or secondary tumours, infections, inflammatory arthritides, metabolic bone disease, and visceral and vascular disorders (all of which are comparatively uncommon causes of chronic back pain) have been excluded, then we are left with the rather vague diagnosis of 'non-specific low back pain' or 'mechanical back pain'. These labels do no more than to emphasize our poor understanding of the causes. There is usually pain across the lower lumbar region, particularly at the L5–S1 level. However, there is often pain or paraesthesia radiating into the buttock or down the leg in the typical 'sciatica' distribution, even though there is no evidence of compression of the lumbar or sacral nerve roots.

This pain may be caused by disorders in several spinal structures. The articular joints of the spine—the apophyseal or facet joints—are as prone to degenerative changes as any other joints. They are innervated by branches of the posterior rami of the spinal nerves whose anterior primary rami are the roots of the major cutaneous nerves of the lower trunk and legs. It is possible, therefore, that pain arising in these joints may be referred in the distribution of the subcutaneous nerves and be experienced as pain in the lower back and limbs. When these joints become degenerate they form bony outgrowths which may reduce the diameter of intervertebral foraminae, so compressing the nerve roots and their associated sheaths. This can cause pain which is felt in the distribution of these nerves. Deterioration of the elasticity and volume of intervertebral discs normally happens with ageing, but it may also be particularly marked following trauma or surgery to the discs, and it imposes new strains on the facet joints. These joints are not normally weight bearing, but the new stresses may make them function abnormally and cause pain.

When there has been compression of nerve roots by demonstrable disc pathology, the pain and dysfunction of the nerve may persist even when compression has been surgically relieved. Prolonged compression of nervous tissue results in permanent damage and just as motor function may remain impaired (causing a foot drop or even urinary incontinence) then sensory impairment may become permanent. This can result in numbness, paraesthesia, abnormal sensations such as burning or stabbing pain, or constant aching pain. Not all of these pains felt in the distribution of nerve roots have the characteristics of nerve-damage pain (aching pain is more characteristic of muscle and joint pain) and some of these pains probably have a mixed origin. Certainly long-term painful stimulation of muscles and joints as well as abnormal function of damaged nerves may result in long-term changes in activity in the nerve cells of the spinal cord. These changes result in the perception of pain in response to normal mechanical stimuli and an enhanced sensitivity of the peripheral structures (see Chapter 2).

Most patients with back pain have some tenderness over the back muscles. This may be associated with muscle spasm, for example following acute back injuries. Increased tenderness of muscles is part of the spread of hypersensitivity that develops around an area of injury, but in some cases the muscle pain may be the primary source of pain. Primary fibromyalgia commonly involves the back muscles resulting in widespread pain and stiffness with no evidence of an underlying skeletal or neurological problem. Local myofascial trigger points producing local and referred pain may be a primary soft tissue problem or a reaction to underlying injury.

Neck pain

Neck pain shares many of the features of back pain. Acute injuries may result from trauma causing disc prolapse with consequent compression of nerve roots and pain referred to the distribution of those nerves. As well as neck pain this will usually produce pain in the arm (brachialgia). More usually neck pain does not involve disc prolapse. The so-called whiplash injury, caused by the sudden acceleration of a car being hit from behind, is mostly a soft tissue injury with ligamentous sprain. The normal course is for healing to occur over a period of weeks, but in some patients the pain persists with marked tenderness of the posterior neck muscles and restriction of normal movements long after the injury would be expected to have healed. This may represent a form of myofascial syndrome and, as is frequently seen in this condition, referred pain and paraesthesiae in the arms may lead to the erroneous belief that there is compression of nerve roots.

Degenerative changes in the cervical spine are almost as common as in the lumbar spine. Reduction of disc height, osteophytes, and facet joint arthritis all contribute to the picture of cervical spondylosis. Although there is sometimes demonstrable compression of cervical nerves in this condition, in most instances the pain felt as occipital headache or in the arm.

Management of chronic back pain

There is no treatment for chronic back pain that will consistently prove effective. As the cause is usually poorly understood, it is difficult to be specific about treatment. Most forms of treatment recommended for back pain will be effective sometimes, and often when specific causes for pain have been eliminated or dealt with it is appropriate to work through a range of less specific therapies until one is found to be helpful. However, certain general principles are important. Prolonged immobility is generally deleterious in chronic back and neck pain, so bed rest and the continual wearing of corsets and collars are harmful. Immobility results in weakness and shortening of muscles, and immobile joints become stiff and painful on movement.

Treatment for chronic back pain should be explained to the patient as being an active process and not a passive treatment. Most therapies will at best help to relieve some of the pain for a time. This should be seen as part of a rehabilitation process, enabling and encouraging a gradual improvement in mobility and fitness with a graded programme of increasing activity. Exercise programmes may not directly reduce pain, but increased range of movement, muscle strength, and mobility improve the ability to cope with chronic pain and reduce disability. Many patients equate pain with disability and it is important to reduce this association if there is to be some improvement in the quality of life. Reducing 'pain behaviour', improving the cognitive aspects of chronic pain, and helping the patient to become less helpless as a result of their pain are important aspects of the management of chronic back pain.

Manipulation

During manipulation of the spine the vertebrae are moved beyond their normal physiological range of movement, but within their anatomical range. Several schools of manipulation have developed outside conventional medicine, although many of the techniques are now recognized by the medical profession as being of benefit. The differences in theory, diagnostic methods, and manipulative technique between such schools as chiropractic, osteopathy, and the Maitland school of physiotherapy are beyond the scope of this book, but they all aim to relieve pain by restoring normal spinal mobility and function. Manipulators move vertebral bodies either directly or indirectly by traction and twisting actions.

There is no doubt that many patients with chronic back or neck pain benefit from this type of treatment, especially when it is applied periodically over a prolonged time. Results often compare favourably with more conventional hospital treatments. Patients should only be referred to professionally trained practitioners who only use manipulative techniques where appropriate, and who can recognize when medical advice is necessary.

Medication

Drugs will not cure back pain. Most patients with chronic back pain consume medication which is of little benefit and merely serves to give them the feeling that they are 'doing something'. Some drugs may help the patient to relax more comfortably and to achieve more mobility.

NSAIDs may be useful in the short- to medium-term management of back pain. They can act as analgesics even when there is no continuing inflammatory process. However, they are not always well tolerated by patients and are not without hazards (see Chapter 5). A long acting anti-inflammatory analgesic taken before going to bed will help many patients who have difficulty in obtaining a comfortable night's sleep or awake stiff and in pain.

The use of opioid drugs in the management of chronic back pain is controversial. Most patients attending pain clinics are taking or have tried one of the mild opioid drugs such as dextropropoxyphene or dihydrocodeine, usually in combination with paracetamol. They may consume these in increasing doses in a desperate attempt to obtain relief, risking an overdose of paracetamol. These weak opioids have a tendency to become habit forming and cause a mild abstinence syndrome if withdrawn.

Strong opioids such as morphine and methadone carry the medical and social stigma of addictive potential and their effect on mood may be more obvious than their analgesic properties in chronic pain. In fact, chronic back pain, in common with much chronic pain, often responds poorly to opioid analgesics. This may reflect its neurogenic and behavioural components as opposed to the nociceptive aspects. Some patients do have an opioid-responsive component of their pain and, although these drugs rarely produce complete relief, they may reduce the intensity of pain enough to improve mobility and enable patients to participate in some of life's activities from which they are otherwise excluded.

The prescription of analgesic drugs should be carefully considered. There must be demonstrable improvement in pain control with acceptable side-effects. If pain control cannot be shown to have improved objectively then there is no justification for continuing analgesic therapy. However, if these drugs can improve the quality of life, there is perhaps no justification for not prescribing them. These arguments apply to both weak and strong opioid analgesics. Weak analgesics may be sufficient and are not subject to such extensive medical supervision and legal controls. However, their low ceiling of therapeutic effect means that increasing the dose increases side-effects whilst rarely increasing benefits. A small dose of strong opioid may be more effective and cause fewer problems than a large dose of weak opioid. It is generally believed that strong opioid drugs should only be prescribed for chronic pain (with a normal life expectancy) in a few restricted circumstances. Their use is thought to be justified only when all other measures to relieve pain have been found inadequate, when a clear improvement in the quality of life can be demonstrated, when major behavioural problems and drug abuse tendencies have been excluded, and when the advantages and disadvantages of such treatment have been carefully discussed with the patient.

If strong opioid drugs are prescribed, the first choice must be a long-acting preparation of morphine, taken regularly. Shorter acting drugs such as pethidine or dipipanone are more likely to lead to 'demand consumption' and escalating dose, as the short-term euphoriant effect becomes more important than the analgesia. Withdrawal may also be much more of a problem with these drugs. It must be stressed that there are relatively few sufferers from chronic back pain who are likely to benefit from this type of analgesia.

Antidepressants and anticonvulsants　Back pain may be caused by continued activation of nociceptors. However, analgesic drugs which usually help relieve nociceptive pain are frequently only of very limited benefit in back pain. This must mean that much of the pain is not arising from peripheral nociception. Stress and anxiety as well as behavioural changes can contribute to the experience of pain, and there is often an element of neurogenic pain. This arises from damage to peripheral nerve tissue or spinal cord, or from abnormal function within the spinal cord resulting from previous damage. This type of pain may respond more to drugs which have a modulating effect on nerve function and the pain perception process (see Chapter 11).

The tricyclic antidepressants may be helpful in this context. Their mode of action is not fully understood but the enhancement of nor-adrenergic and serotoninergic mechanisms in the CNS seems to be important. The drugs have a direct analgesic effect on neurogenic pain, and lessen anxiety and depression which commonly accompany chronic back pain. A single night-time dose will provide a restful sleep for patients whose pain and anxiety prevent adequate rest. Amitriptyline is the drug most frequently used in this situation although other tricyclics such as dothiepin are useful if the side-effects of amitriptyline cannot be tolerated. The dose providing pain relief is often less than is needed for depression, and the analgesic effect of tricyclics seems to be separate from their anti-depressant properties.

Anticonvulsants have long been used in the management of neurogenic pain, and are most useful for the lancinating or 'electric shock' type of pain. Alone, or in combination with a tricyclic antidepressant, drugs such as carbamazepine, sodium valproate or clonazepam can be effective in reducing sharp shooting pains which sometimes follow damage to the peripheral or the central nervous system.

Injection treatment

Invasive treatments for chronic back pain rarely produce permanent relief, but there are situations where some form of injection treatment may be helpful. Chronic back and leg pain is unlikely to be the result of inflammatory change around nerve roots, and yet some patients with long-term pain seem to gain substantial relief from the injection of local anaesthetic and steroid into the epidural space. The mechanism is unknown, but it has been postulated that the injections cause breakdown of adhesions and scar tissue, or relieve pressure on nerve tissue by producing some necrosis of epidural fat. The pain may return after many months, but if the period of relief is substantial, it seems to be worth repeating the procedure periodically.

Injection of steroid into the spinal apophyseal joints (facet joints) relieves chronic back pain in some patients. It seems to be most effective when there is evidence of arthritis in these joints, when pain is particularly associated with extension and twisting movements of the spine, and when pain is worse on prolonged sitting or standing. The mechanism is obscure and unfortunately, like most treatments for back pain, it is difficult to prove the benefits objectively or even reliably to predict outcome. It may be possible to produce equally good results from injections placed around the outside of the joint capsule and lesions made at a variety of sites in the posterior compartment of the spine. Any relief of pain may last from a few weeks to a year or more. For patients who do experience prolonged relief the procedure is worth repeating. Similar results may be obtained by producing a lesion in the nerves supplying the joints using a needle positioned under radiological control and passing a high frequency current (radiofrequency) through the tip. However, results of such destructive procedures may be no better than simple injections.

Injections of local anaesthetic, with or without steroid, or stimulation with acupuncture needles may relieve back pain when it is found to be associated with painful tense bands in the muscles. Myofascial pain seems to be a frequent component of back pain and desensitization of trigger points may provide some reduction of pain.

All these invasive techniques may produce a period of partial relief from chronic back pain which then allows more active involvement in rehabilitation programmes. They are rarely a long-term solution but may help in the overall management of the chronic back pain sufferer.

Back school

Many physiotherapy departments provide a back school. This may be held as a single session or a longer course in which patients are taught about spinal mechanics, correct ways of moving, lifting, sitting, and lying. They are also offered a programme of back-strengthening exercises. The emphasis is on preventing further deterioration of back problems by maintaining fitness and correct posture.

Psychological management

The personal psychological effects related to loss of self-esteem and chronic disability, and the resulting effects on family, social, and financial aspects of life all contribute to the long-term suffering and interfere with the rehabilitation of many back pain sufferers. Long-term managment must attend to these aspects of the condition as well as aiming to improve function and mobility. A pain management programme with input from a clinical psychologist, a physiotherapist, and an occupational therapist can be an important aspect of helping the patient to cope with their physical and psychological problems effectively and to move away from the purely medical model of finding a 'cure' for back pain (see Chapter 3).

Further reading

Cailliet, M. D. (1981). *Low back pain syndrome*. Davis, Philadelphia.
Parker, H. and Main, C. J. (1990). *Living with back pain*. Manchester University Press.
Key, S. (1991). *Back in action*. Century, London.

11 *Neurogenic pain*

Pain and damage to the nervous system
Why neurogenic pain arises
Incidence of pain in disease of the CNS
Iatrogenic causes
Opioid responsiveness and resistance
Use of antidepressants and anticonvulsants
TENS

The nervous system acts as a whole, from the upper motor neuron to the endplate on flexor digiti minimi, and from the sensory receptor in the little toe to the sensory cortex. Among its vital functions is damage detection and avoidance. This intricate and integrated function is the reason for pain perception.

Thus all pain is perceived through nervous system function. Disorder in the nervous system is likely to result in a failure of the ability to distinguish between non-pain normality and the damage signal perceived as pain. An abnormality in nervous system function that can result in pain being perceived where no tissue damage exists can start anywhere between the receptor and the cortex.

Pain and damage to the nervous system

We do not yet know enough of receptor function to understand if an abnormality at this level can result in pain. It is becoming clear that immune cells have receptors for the endogenous opioid ligands and that the reception and onward transmission of noxious stimulation can be modulated at this level. Receptors are sensitized by the substances released by tissue damage. It is thus extremely likely that receptor abnormalities exist which result in the perception of pain in the absence of noxious stimulation. This may be partially responsible for allodynia—the sensation of pain in response to harmless stimulation.

The mechanism behind the pain of sympathetic dystrophy, or causalgia, is not understood. It may be the result of axonal abnormality. However, in animal models it appears that pain can be generated by the presence of adrenalin at sensory receptors when there has been nerve damage, and that this may be responsible for some of the features of this syndrome.

It is certain that damage to peripheral nerve fibres will cause pain. When a sensory nerve is divided the area that it supplies becomes numb, and then axons in the distal end atrophy. Axons sprout from the proximal end, enter the distal end (if it is close), and grow down, eventually re-innervating it. If the cut ends are not well aligned some of these sprouts emerge from the sides of the join instead of growing down the distal end. These sprouts develop intensely sensitive mechanoceptor terminals which cause pain when stimulated. If there is no distal end for the sprouts to grow down, they will form a neuroma, which will be intensely sensitive and painful.

Why neurogenic pain arises

Once a sensory nerve enters the CNS at the dorsal horn of the spinal cord the signals that it is transmitting are subjected to a system of controls. Incoming information that has no significance is filtered out so that what is perceived is relevant. There is continuous traffic up all the fibres in sensory nerves including the smallest that carry pain information. Unless tissue is about to be damaged, this incoming information must be filtered, otherwise an uncontrolled and unbearable barrage of information would reach consciousness.

Incidence of pain in disease of the CNS

Disease of the CNS is not uncommon. For example, there are 100 000 strokes in the UK each year. Two per cent of these give rise to post-stroke pain (which used to be known as the thalamic syndrome) so there are 2000 new cases of this every year. Three per cent of the population have multiple sclerosis, of whom half have chronic pain. In half of these, the pain is of central origin. It is unfortunate that the incidence of these pains is not widely known. There is no cure for most diseases of the CNS, so once a diagnosis is made patients are often left to suffer and told nothing more can be done. Sufferers frequently (and mistakenly) believe that they are unique in suffering from pain caused by their condition, and this belief adds to their distress.

Iatrogenic causes

Disease can damage nervous tissue, but so can attempts to treat it. Patients who continue to suffer from back pain following spinal surgery may have the typical features of a neurogenic pain—it is burning in character, has a stabbing element, and is associated with loss of pin-prick sensation or allodynia. If these alterations and the pain were present before surgery then they must be due to nerve damage caused by the disease for which the operation was performed. But if the pain has altered from a nocigenic pain to a neurogenic pain since the operation was done, it must result from nerve damage caused by the surgery.

Destructive lesions in the nervous system are still made to provide pain relief (see Chapter 8). They relieve pain for a while, but eventually cause a deafferentation pain, resulting from interference with sensory function. This pain is extremely unpleasant, often worse than the pain that the patient had before the lesion was made. Although central and peripheral nervous system lesions have been made for many years we do not know their success rate or the complication rate, or the incidence of deafferentation pain. It is possible that a valuable means of providing long-term pain relief is now being neglected. On the other hand, the complication rate may be so high that the use of these treatments can never be justified.

Opioid responsiveness and resistance

The use of opioid drugs in pain control is controversial in many situations (see Chapter 5), and neurogenic pain is one of these. Opiates interfere with the perception of pain by inhibiting onward transmission from the outer layers of the grey matter of the dorsal horn of the spinal cord. They also alter mood and cause drowsiness which must alter a sufferer's perception of pain. Pain caused by an alteration in sensory processing as a result of damage to the CNS should not respond to opioid analgesia, because it is generated proximal to the outer laminae of the dorsal horn. However, some people with typical neurogenic pain do seem to get some relief from drugs in this group. Is this relief due to the more central effects of these drugs? If so, does this matter? If the drug gives relief and the patient does not abuse it, the patient must be better off with it than without it. It is important not to let prejudice interfere with humanity.

Use of antidepressants and anticonvulsants

Neurogenic pain results from uncontrolled sensory nervous system activity. It is either generated from sprouts from damaged axons or as a result of reduced inhibitory controls. Drugs which affect over-excitability of neuronal activity are more likely to be effective against this pain than drugs that block or reduce input from sensory receptors into the CNS. Analgesics reduce the amount of incoming information either by reducing the stimulation of nociceptor nerve terminals, or by blocking the input from nociceptor nerve fibres into the spinal cord.

General anaesthetics act by reducing the activity of the whole nervous system to such an extent that there is no perception of any incoming information. Local anaesthetics have the same effect, but selectively. Although these are the most powerful analgesics they could not be used in pain management because of their effect on function. What are needed are drugs that reduce central nervous function while allowing normal activity to continue.

The drugs used to control epilepsy and the antidepressant drugs meet these requirements. The first use of such a drug for neurogenic pain was the use of carbamazepine in trigeminal neuralgia. It made a dramatic difference to a condition which has all the characteristics of both peripheral and central sensory nervous system instability. It is lancinating, extremely severe, of short duration and triggered by peripheral stimulation.

The use of the tricyclic antidepressant amitriptyline with carbamazepine in post-herpetic neuralgia soon followed. Since then amitriptyline has been shown to be superior to placebo in a variety of neurogenic pains.

Neurogenic pain often responds to drugs such as these in lower doses than are used for treating epilepsy or depression. It is best to start with the smallest dose available, such as 10 mg amitriptyline at night and 100 mg carbamazepine once a day. The dosage is then increased at a rate tolerable for the patient, until either the pain is reduced or side-effects have become unacceptable. If one drug in a class has no effect, it is worthwhile trying another. Clomipramine, desipramine, and nortriptyline have been successful alternatives to one another, although the newer serotonin re-uptake inhibitors have been disappointing. Similarly, if carbamazepine causes side-effects or is ineffective, sodium valproate or clonazepam should be tried.

TENS

A barrage of non-painful sensation from TENS may block neurogenic pain. TENS can also enhance the effect of anticonvulsants and tricyclics. To make TENS as effective as possible the electrodes must be put over areas where sensation is intact. If stimulation seems to make the pain worse the electrodes should be moved. This is as harmless a way of relieving pain as can be found, so it is worth taking pains to make it effective.

Index